Stronger Together:

A Couple's Guide to Navigating Your Relationship After Baby

by Zara Arshad, MSc., MFT, RP, PMH-C

Stronger Together: A Couple's Guide to Navigating Your Relationship After Baby

by Zara Arshad, MSc., MFT, RP, PMH-C
Registered Psychotherapist
Certified Perinatal Mental Health Specialist

Liability Disclaimer

For more information and other queries, contact: connect@myottawatherapist.com

Dedication

This is dedicated to new parents who are trying to work through challenges in their relationship while learning to become parents for the first time. To all the couples working hard to improve their relationship with courage and resilience. To my clients who have allowed me the privilege of helping them while also continuously teaching me about life and relationships. Last, but not the least, to my husband and my children. Without your love, patience, and unwavering support, this book would not be possible. I am so grateful for you in my life!

Table of Contents

Introduction

If you are reading this, chances are you have made a decision to invest in the growth of your relationship. As a therapist who specializes in supporting couples navigating their relationship postpartum, I am passionate about helping couples like you develop healthy and secure relationships. While I have written this book for new parents, the contents of this book are relevant to anyone who is in a committed relationship and interested in learning how to improve as a couple.

Before you begin reading the sections in this book, I want to share that I wrote this book keeping my readers in mind who may be new parents. I am aware of the fact you may lack the time and energy needed to read a comprehensive book. For this reason, I have not covered everything there is to know about a couple's relationship. Rather, I have written about topics that I hope bring the most amount of value to you as you learn to navigate your relationship through the transition into parenthood, or as you await the arrival of your precious baby.

As we move forward on this journey together, it is a privilege to be a part of your relationship's healing and growth. When you begin the reading and exercises, some of this may feel new and challenging. As you reconnect to yourself and your partner or spouse, there will be moments of vulnerability you may not have experienced within your partnership before. I understand this process, not only in my clinical professional role, but also in my personal role as a wife and a mother.

I can't tell you why I do what I do without sharing the fact that my parents are divorced. I grew up in a dysfunctional family system which did not provide stability or security. While this had a hand in shaping me into who I am today, it also had a hand in pulling me towards the mental health field. As I grew older and understood the world better, I felt a natural desire to help other individuals and families who may also be struggling.

Fast forward to when I had my own children, I became particularly interested in wanting to help young couples. My interest in young couples began after experiencing postpartum challenges and marital distress of my own. After I gave birth to my sweet son in 2017, I was fortunate to not experience any postpartum mood disorder. I did, however, experience several mental health struggles in the first six months postpartum.

There were many rough days and nights with mixed feelings and tears. My husband couldn't understand or relate; therefore, he did not know how to help me in the way I needed during those first few months. I felt alone in my physical and emotional pain. I also felt dumbfounded, wondering why nobody had prepared me for this. There was plenty of medical information and physical health resources made available to me, such as follow-up appointments with my doctor, perinatal massages, physiotherapy, yoga, birthing, labor, and breastfeeding classes, and postpartum mommy/baby classes.

But what about postpartum mental health? I did not receive much information on this topic, nor was I provided any resources, nor was there any support forthcoming from anyone around me or in the community.

And then came our adorable daughter in April of 2020. My husband and I struggled in our relationship more than we had after our first child was born. Not only were we parents to a toddler and a newborn, we were also in the start of a global pandemic, completely isolated with no help or break from being parents. As time went on, we found ourselves spinning around, trying to get through each day...and just like that, days turned into weeks, and weeks turned into months.

We came to a point where we realized that even though we were physically together more than usual, emotionally we were drifting further apart.

From both of my postpartum experiences, I became increasingly aware of two things:

1) There is an incredible lack of mental health support or resources readily available to expecting couples and new parents.

2) It is vitally important for the couple's relationship to be a source of stability, love, and safety for children.

I knew our marriage had to be the main source of all things good for our children. Our relationship needed to be strong, happy, safe, committed, secure, stable, and connected for our children to feel all those things inside of them. From this place of awareness, I have become passionate about helping other young couples who are either thinking of having children, currently expecting, or have children already.

Through this book, I want to provide enough inspiration, guidance, and practical tools for young couples to feel the push towards strengthening and improving their partnership in the hopes that the tiny beings they wish to bring into their lives are raised in emotionally secure homes. I also hope to encourage couples to strive for healing, improvement, and growth—not perfection. Modeling healthy behavior during or after moments of distress is far more useful than modeling perfection to your children.

I am all too aware how caring for babies or small children and having inadequate sleep can make it difficult for you to learn, retain, and absorb new information. Therefore, I have provided space for your thoughts at the end of each chapter to make it easy for you to remember tools and strategies, and to motivate you to implement the concepts in this book. I encourage you and your partner to jot down notes which can serve as reminders and actionable steps for practicing what you are learning. At the same time, I want to stress the importance of using your judgment before carrying out any ideas presented. This book contains many helpful suggestions, but they are not one-size-fits-all. Even when circumstances are similar, relationships are unique.

I encourage you to trust your intuition and only implement those ideas that feel safe to try in your relationship. If the concepts don't feel safe, or you need additional support, I recommend seeking individual or couple's therapy. This book is not meant to be a replacement for psychotherapy, nor is it meant to be counseling advice.

Finally, in writing this book, my sincere hope is to create an opportunity for couples to have thoughtful conversations and experience meaningful changes as they increase understanding of one another, improve communication, and deepen their connection. I thank you for the trust in allowing me to guide this part of your journey...let's begin!

Warmly,

Zara

Finding Us

Before we start, I will share a poem which beautifully captures the spirit of this book. It is written by Jessica Urlichs, mother and best-selling author of poetry books on early motherhood. The poem is titled "Finding Us" and it is from her book, *From One Mom to a Mother* (2020):

> I would often hear how much closer you'd become in your relationship after having children.
> I'd see the fabricated newborn photos behind smiles and perfect lighting, engorged breasts and awkward poses.
> I know, because I have them.
> But it's the part in between you becoming closer that isn't talked about much.
> The confusing part.
>
> Where the love of the child you've created fuses you together but can also be the very thing that holds you at arm's length.
>
> Where all of a sudden your love for each other inexplicably takes a turn for a greater more powerful love that you've never felt before and you accept it, before really being able to process it.
>
> Where you look at each other over the piles of laundry, breast pumps, dishes, nappies, ointments and the distance between you feels like an obstacle course of cumbersome chores and challenges.
>
> Where your hands slide past each other's to hold on to smaller ones.
> Where you're told to nurture your relationship, but not how to, when in reality the only place for it right now comes last.
>
> Where we have made ourselves smaller in this new picture, stripped down in its unfiltered format.

We don't talk about that part.
The raw and exposed part that grounds you to the core but also holds you in a state of shock.
Just constant, and no need to align that word to anything.
Because that's what it is.
Constant.

I asked myself, what now?
It wasn't the deep and meaningful chat I thought we needed.
Because this journey we're on, is that, every day, even without words.
Instead it was the on the surface stuff, the new pieces we were picking out and rearranging around each other. The favourite movie chat, the bad jokes, the light behind the tired eyes that comes with newfound discovery.
The fun light-hearted stuff.
It was going from living and breathing each other in our most non sheltered state, to putting on some makeup, nice but old clothes, and sitting across from one another at a restaurant and making the effort to know each other again.
The small things, the things that still matter.
It's a new introduction.
No one talks about that.

Chapter 1: *The Fourth Trimester*

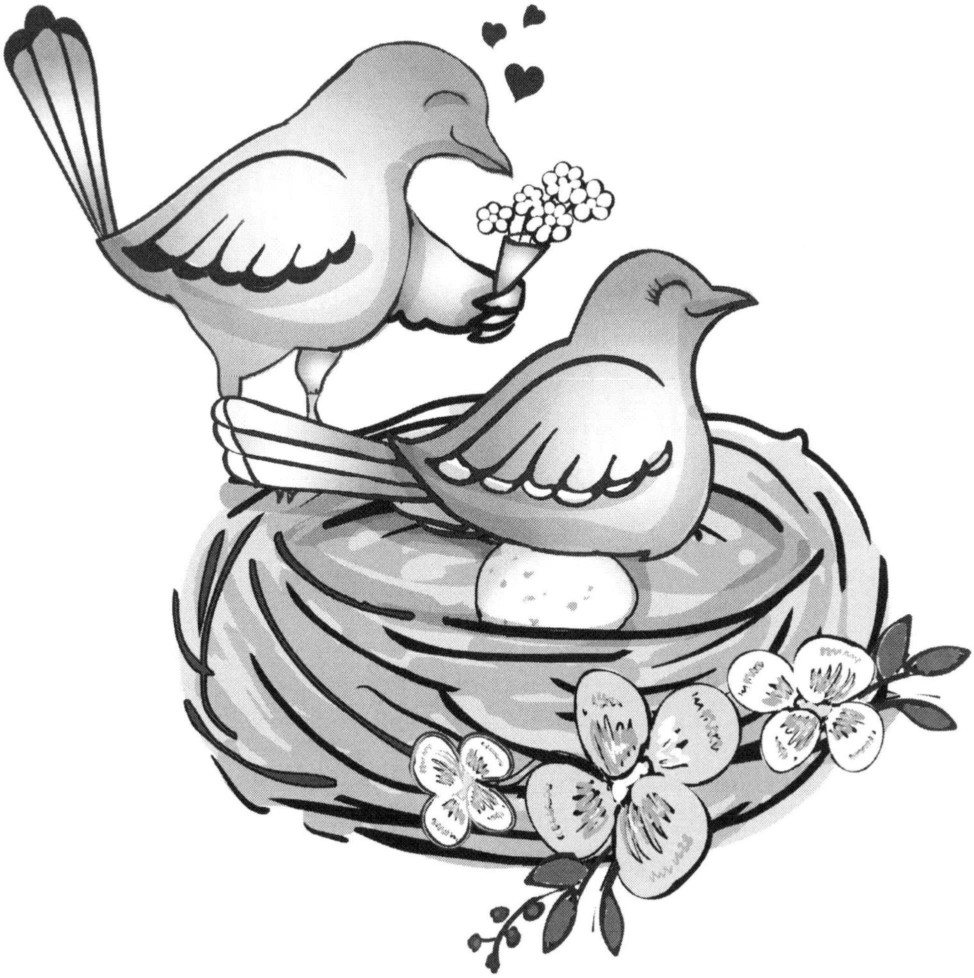

What to Expect

Having a baby typically is associated with feelings of happiness, joy, and pride across societies and cultures. And why not? It is the start of a beautiful journey and a special time in a couple's life, especially for those who struggle with years of infertility. Many couples dream about the time they will hold their little baby in their arms, all bundled up, snuggled in, and sleeping. Others think about having an adorable baby with a gummy smile crawling around the house. Yet others envision the first time their baby will reach out with their tiny arms and say, "mama" or "dada." While there are so many heart-melting reasons to be overjoyed and in love when your baby is born, there are also many reasons why couples struggle with other emotions after the birth of their child. Unfortunately, these emotions are less talked about and less understood among couples, or in societies in general.

My husband and I were overjoyed to find out we were expecting. We were excited, nervous, happy, and so grateful during the pregnancy. While these feelings carried on for us after having our son, I also experienced several challenges which caused feelings of guilt, sadness, resentment, anger, and confusion. I will share a little about my experience from the first few months postpartum to give some context to those feelings that I had.

I felt heavy, and I ached everywhere the first five days after my son was born, as though a car had hit me head-on. My body was painfully sore from laboring thirty-three hours. My feet were swollen like balloons, and each step I took gave me a painful reminder of the stitches I had. I will spare you other details of the physical recovery, but let's just say the first month postpartum was not a fun ride.

When it came to physical recovery, I found there to be plenty of information, resources, and products available to help me (well, sometimes) for my aches and pains. However, when it came to my mental health, I did not consider I might need support because my attention was focused intensely on my son. In retrospect, my mental health was not in the forefront of my mind even as a therapist, nor was it a topic ever brought up around me in perinatal classes or medical appointments.

In juggling the tasks of new motherhood, my own mental health fell to the wayside. As a result, it was the emotional recovery that caught me the most off guard. And the worst part was I didn't know who to turn to for help.

I tried turning to my husband once for support about three weeks postpartum, when I shared my frustrations, anger, helplessness, and uncertainty around breastfeeding. I remember trying to communicate all of this late at night over a screaming baby who was struggling to feed at that very moment. Meanwhile, I was crying because I was in physical pain and discomfort from the injuries of birth. This was 21 days of me trying to feed my son and feeling like I was failing miserably.

I was exhausted.

I was drained.

I was at my wits' end.

As my husband and I stepped into an angry exchange of words that night, I felt pathetic. I felt this way because I could not figure out the very basics of feeding my child. I thought to myself, *I am the mother, I am supposed to nourish my son, then why can't I figure it out?!*

Looking back now, I think I also felt weak and vulnerable in that moment as a woman trying to explain my struggles to a man, albeit my husband, who could not understand or relate in any way. My helplessness in the situation made me resent my husband and, at times, made me angry with my son. This only fueled my feelings of guilt and sadness for not being able to feed him.

That night, the outcome of the conversation with my husband was not what I had hoped. It was hardly a conversation, considering how frustrated I was trying to explain myself over my son's inconsolable crying all the while dealing with my physical pain and discomfort. My kind-hearted husband felt helpless and frustrated himself as he could not relate to my struggles or my pain and did not know how to help me. It was late at night, we were both exhausted, and my son would not stop crying. I walked away feeling hurt, doubting myself even more as a woman and a mother. I felt more alone than ever before. I felt isolated in my pain, my frustrations, my doubts, and my sadness.

I did not believe that I could talk to any of my friends because I was the first one to have a child. They wouldn't have known how to comfort and support me in ways I needed. I couldn't talk to my family because I didn't feel comfortable being vulnerable with them at the time.

It would be untrue for me to say my husband and I did not have help. In fact, we were fortunate to have parents and siblings taking turns visiting us and helping during the first three months postpartum. However, speaking for myself, what I lacked was emotional support. In hindsight, I needed it as much as I needed physical support. I did not know this at the time because no one really prepares an expecting mother by talking about the emotional challenges that occur in the fourth trimester—and beyond.

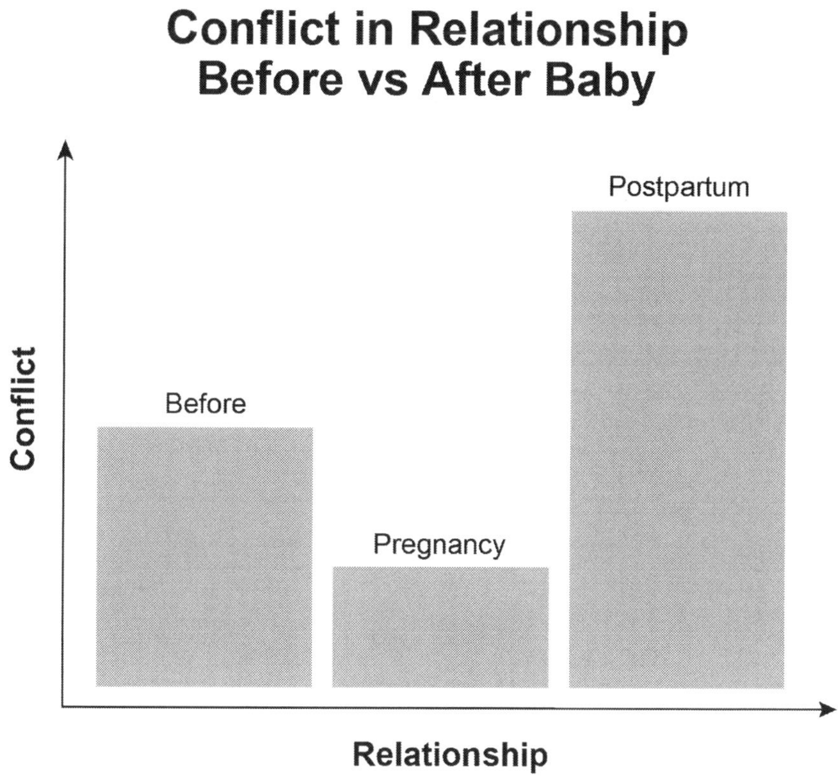
Conflict in Relationship
Before vs After Baby
Conflict
Before
Pregnancy
Postpartum
Relationship

I ask myself now, Why is that? Why are expecting couples not told about the realities of life after baby? Why are couples deprived of the knowledge they need beforehand in order to prepare their relationship and safeguard their mental health?

That night—the night I had an argument with my husband—I googled a question about breastfeeding during the third, fourth, or fifth feed of the night (I usually lost count after the third feed). My husband slept peacefully next to me, oblivious to his son being awake for the umpteenth time. If you're a mother, you know exactly how I felt watching my husband sleep! In my search for answers on how to breastfeed a baby who is struggling to latch, I stumbled upon an online community of mothers reaching out to one another for answers and support for their postpartum struggles.

Over the next few months, I read dozens upon dozens of stories all similar to my own, and some stories were more painful than my own. I poured through the questions and comments from mothers around the world, all discussing their physical, mental, and emotional struggles. Many were even discussing dissatisfaction with their partner. I remember for many weeks, my routine became to scroll through the comments all night long as I fed my son. I found comfort, support, and so much strength by reading the words of these mothers. Thanks to this online community, I finally didn't feel alone. I felt normal in my struggles. I felt hope.

This newfound sense of belonging, normalcy, and hope gave me strength and courage to look at myself as a capable mother. I started to feel more confident in my abilities, I became more compassionate towards myself, and I felt motivated to try new things and do the best I could for my son.

I share my first postpartum experience not to scare any of you who may be new parents or expecting your baby, rather, to enlighten you so you don't feel alone as I did when you face your challenges. My sincere desire is to validate the challenges you may be going through or you may face in the future. My hope is that every new mother and their spouse or partner understands they are not alone in their struggles.

As this section comes to a close, here are five lessons I learned from my first postpartum experience which I want to share with you:

1. It is completely normal to struggle mentally and emotionally after giving birth. It is normal to have self-doubts. It is normal to feel sad. It is normal to feel frustrated with yourself, your partner, and even your baby. It is normal to experience guilt after feeling frustrated. It is normal to have breakdowns. It is normal to experience anger. It is all so normal.

2. You are not the only one feeling the things you're feeling and thinking the things you're thinking. Chances are every parent at some point has had the exact same thoughts or feelings as you.

3. If you are a new mother, your partner is also a new parent. Even if your partner has a child from a previous relationship, they are still in new territory as a co-parent with you. Which means they may not know what to expect and what to do. Your partner may not understand or relate to what you're experiencing, so how can they be expected to support you in exactly the way you need? This is not to make you feel alone, rather, to help you manage your expectations of those around you who may not know what you're going through. In later chapters, I will teach you communication tools to help you share your expectations with your partner so you can enlist their support.

4. It is so important to reach out to other parents in your life and talk about what you're experiencing. Don't only focus on talking about the upside or share cute baby pictures. Talk about what is difficult, what hurts, and what impacts your mental health. I believe we need to start creating a culture where it becomes normal and encouraged to be transparent about mental health and relationship challenges as new parents.

5. It is easy to lose yourself in caring for your baby. However, you can only take care of your baby as well as you are taking care of yourself. If you are drained, exhausted, unhappy, and racked with doubts, fears, frustrations, questions, and guilt, how effective will you be in caring for your child? In later chapters, I will teach you practical and effective ways in which you can take care of yourself while caring for your baby.

Now, let's take a look at relevant and helpful topics for couples navigating their relationship after baby through my lens as a therapist.

Mood Disturbances

In recent times, postpartum mood disorders have received more attention and acknowledgement in Western society. This recognition is important in ensuring that women don't suffer alone and are provided adequate mental health support in the form of talk therapy and/or prescribed medication. Before I discuss postpartum mood any further, it is important to differentiate between a postpartum mood disorder and the baby blues.

The Diagnostic and Statistical Manual of Mental Disorders (5th ed.; DSM–5; American Psychiatric Association, 2013), a manual used among health care professionals in many parts of the world for diagnosing mental health disorders, gives limited recognition to perinatal mental health. Furthermore, there is a significant gap between the criteria specified by the DSM-5 for receiving a perinatal diagnosis and what researchers, clinicians, and other professionals in the field of perinatal mental health believe the criteria should be (Segre & Davis, 2013). Therefore, I will share my observations as a clinician working with the perinatal population to describe some of the differences I have observed between a mood disorder and the baby blues.

A postpartum mood disorder is less common, starts within the first year postpartum, lasts for a prolonged period of time, has a greater impact on a mother's mental health and functioning, and usually does not go away on its own. Baby blues are mood swings that start shortly after birth, are very common, last for a few days or a few weeks, have a lower impact on a mother's mental health and functioning, and usually go away on their own. The following is a list of mixed emotions commonly identified to me by mothers who are experiencing the baby blues:

Anger	Isolation
Anxiety	Joy
Excitement	Loneliness
Fear	Overwhelm
Gratitude	Sadness
Guilt	Worry

If the undesired feelings last more than a few weeks, increase in severity, and diminish your physical and mental functioning, you may be suffering from a postpartum mood disorder.

A mood disorder can impact the birthing parent in various ways, and symptoms can vary from moderate to extreme. Some women may experience it soon after birth, and others may experience it a few months or up to a year after birth. If you are wondering whether you have a mood disorder, you can meet with a professional for an assessment and diagnosis. However, a diagnosis is not a necessary component for managing and improving your mental health. As such, most mothers I work with in my private practice do not come to me with an official diagnosis, nor is it something I need to help them. Realizing you are no longer feeling like yourself and turning to someone for help is more important than fixating on a label.

That being said, a diagnosis can be essential in the following situations: a) you want or need medication, b) your insurance requires it to provide coverage for mental health services rendered, c) you find it helpful to name your struggle in order to understand it better, or d) your symptoms are increasing in severity, and you are attempting or thinking of suicide.

Please note that mental health struggles during pregnancy and postpartum are very common. Having a baby is a huge adjustment and one that requires a lot from you physically, mentally, and emotionally. Hence, it is normal to experience a decline in your mental health. In fact, I prefer to call these mood conditions "disturbances" rather than "disorders" because simply put, a postpartum mood disorder is a temporary disturbance—or a shift—in the way you think, feel, and behave.

The postpartum women I work with in my practice usually report symptoms of depression, anxiety, or both. This is consistent with the findings of a survey on maternal health in Canada (*The Daily*, 2019), where nearly 25 percent of mothers who gave birth in 2018-2019 reported feelings which were consistent with postpartum depression and anxiety. For these reasons, I will only focus on these two mood disturbances in this section.

To help you become familiar with the key characteristics of postpartum depression and postpartum anxiety, I have listed out some of the common thoughts, feelings, and behaviors described to me by new mothers in Figure 1.

Figure 1

Common characteristics found in postpartum depression and postpartum anxiety

	Postpartum Depression:	Postpartum Anxiety:
Thoughts	• "I wish I could go back to my old life." • "It's difficult being a mother." • "Why can't I bond with them?" • "It's my fault. I should know what they need from me." • "I feel like running away from it all." • "I'm not cut out to be a mother."	• "What if they choke on their vomit?" • "I will drop them if I walk down the stairs." • "I'm afraid of leaving them alone." • "I'm afraid of being alone with them." • "I can't do this anymore!" • Disruptive intrusive thoughts
Feelings	• Empty • Guilty • Helpless • Irritable • Overwhelmed • Sad	• Angry • Anxious • Irritable • Out of control • Overwhelmed • Paranoid
Behaviors	• Change in sleeping and eating habits • Frequent crying or emotional withdrawal • Inability to concentrate or remember • Loss of confidence in capabilities • Loss of interest or pleasure in activities • Loss of sexual desire • Withdrawn from partner	• Appearing preoccupied • Change in sleeping and eating habits • Compulsive behaviors • Panic attacks • Focused on planning and structure • Focused on cleaning and organizing • Striving for perfection • Critical of partner

While the table in Figure 1 displays two ends of the spectrum, many postpartum women fall somewhere in between, presenting with symptoms of both depression and anxiety. Some women may suspect their postpartum symptoms are due to an imbalance of hormones, which is possible. If you suspect this is the case, talk to your doctor about your options. If you have attempted to speak to your medical doctor about your postpartum symptoms, and your concerns have been minimized or dismissed, please continue to advocate for yourself and seek out a doctor who will listen to you.

The women who walk into my office largely attribute their symptoms to difficulties related to caring for their baby, managing their relationship with their partner, and transitioning and adjusting to their new role as a mother. These challenges impact their mental health, causing feelings of sadness, anger, resentment, disappointment, fear, anxiety, and more. To demonstrate how mothers present their symptoms to me, I will share Jenn's story:

Jenn came to see me for about six sessions to learn how to manage her anxiety. She reported a history of anxiety since before she had children, but she felt it had worsened since the birth of her second child. As I helped her unpack the anxiety, Jenn shared how angry she was with herself for being critical of her older daughter, Amelia, who was three years old. She shared instances where she would be quick to chide her daughter for not behaving a certain way. At the same time, she was feeling guilty for not being a more loving, carefree mother. Jenn quietly cried as she wondered out loud whether she was a good parent.

She continued to explain her struggles, this time in relation to her marriage. Jenn shared feelings of utter exhaustion taking care of both her children while also taking care of household duties during her maternity leave. To explain what was causing tension in her marriage, Jenn described how she asked her husband to take over the responsibility of Amelia's meals. She sounded visibly upset as she shared how her husband continuously fed their daughter meals that were lacking adequate nutrition, despite Jenn's multiple requests. And to her dismay, he would repeat the same meal several times a week.

She explained feeling extremely bothered by this as it triggered feelings of guilt inside of her for not being able to ensure more nutritious meals for Amelia. This compounded with the guilt she was already experiencing for lacking patience and tenderness with her daughter. Jenn expressed doubts about herself as a mother. She also doubted herself as a wife for frequently lashing out at her husband. Jenn was tired of feeling this way and hated how critical she was towards the people she loved the most. At the same time, she was tired of her husband not listening to her concerns about ensuring adequate nutrition for her children.

With a history of anxiety, conflicting values between her and her husband, relationship distress, negative thought patterns, and feelings of anger, guilt, self-doubt, and self-hatred, it is no wonder Jenn was struggling with a postpartum mood disturbance. As demonstrated by Jenn's story, in my professional experience, I have come to recognize that postpartum mood disturbances are usually triggered when at least two of the following factors are present at the same time:

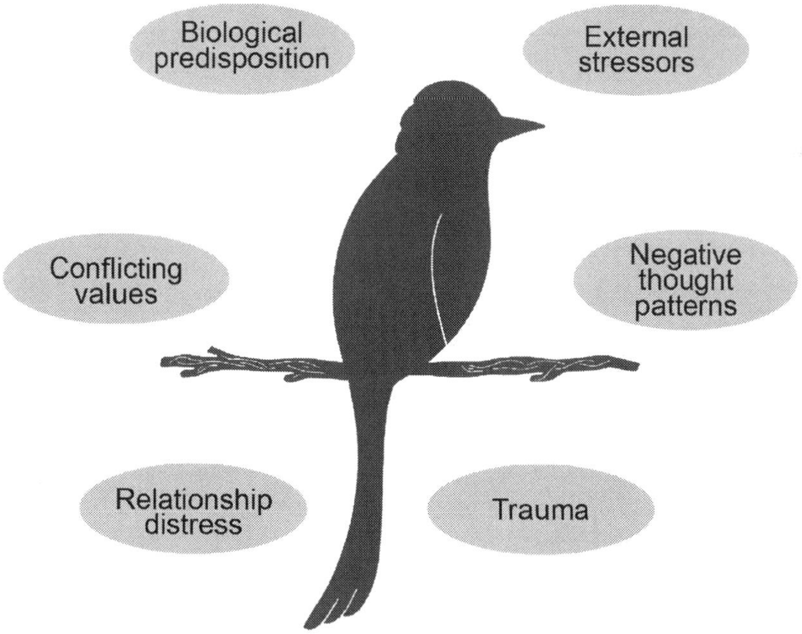
Biological predisposition
External stressors
Conflicting values
Negative thought patterns
Relationship distress
Trauma

1. Biological predisposition: Genetically, you can be predisposed towards depression or anxiety if there is a history in your family of origin.

However, having a family history does not guarantee you will experience a mood disorder. Moreover, women who have a history of depression and anxiety are more likely to experience it after birth (Ghaedrahmati et al., 2017).

2. Negative thought patterns: The thoughts you have towards yourself, another person, or something happening in your environment determine how you feel. If you engage in frequent negative thought patterns, you will frequently experience undesired feelings. Over time, this can lead to feelings of depression, anxiety, or both.

3. Conflicting values: Everyone lives by values that are either spoken or unspoken. Sometimes, a new value you develop can be in conflict with an old value you once had. Other times, values that are important to you can be different from the values that are important to your partner. Still other times, two values can be competing against each other. In all these instances, you will begin to feel confusion, discomfort, and tension if values remain in conflict for a prolonged period of time. I talk about this topic more in-depth in Chapter 4.

4. External stressors: These are factors in your environment that are sometimes in your control and sometimes not. A few examples include: your baby developing a preference for breast and refusing the bottle, involvement of family members or in-laws, lack of sufficient sleep, work-related stress, household duties, conflicting schedules and routines, unemployment, financial stressors, and the need for constant care and attendance towards your baby at the expense of your own needs.

Additionally, the COVID-19 pandemic has been a recent source of significant external stress on expecting and postpartum couples. The increased rate of mental health concerns among postpartum women during the first nine months of the pandemic (Vigod et al., 2021) suggests an increase in postpartum mood disorders since the start of the pandemic.

Some mothers and their partners have experienced increased uncertainty, anxiety, confusion, fear, isolation, and grief due to the loss of their usual coping outlets, community resources, family support, and the loss of experiencing a "normal" pregnancy, delivery, and parental leave.

5. Relationship distress: When one or both partners experience prolonged negative feelings towards the other, such as anger or resentment, it can corrode feelings of mutual connection the couple once shared. This can negatively influence other aspects of their relationship, such as communication, intimacy, and general satisfaction.

6. Trauma: Complications related to infertility, pregnancy, or birth can result in traumatic experiences for women and their partners. The trauma can range from emotional to physical to sexual. Traumatic experiences include:

- Prolonged suffering due to infertility
- Miscarriage(s)
- High-risk pregnancy
- Unwanted pregnancy
- Prolonged sickness and disability during pregnancy
- Re-triggering of previous sexual trauma during medical checkups
- Medical complications at birth
- Laboring and birthing in isolation due to the pandemic
- Unexpected experiences during or after birth, such as the immediate removal of your baby from the birthing room
- Still birth
- Loss after birth
- Not being able to see your baby for weeks if you tested positive for COVID-19
- Social isolation after birth due to the pandemic
- Postpartum complications related to breastfeeding, baby's health, and mother's physical recovery

In some cultures, such as the South Asian culture I belong to, symptoms of a postpartum mood disturbance may not be understood as a mental health concern. Immigrant women from these cultures are more likely to describe their mental health struggles to me as physical symptoms, such as feeling tired or exhausted. These women might also explain away their symptoms by attributing them to missing their family back home or lacking family support to help care for their baby.

If this is you, please know postpartum recovery is not only physical, but also mental and emotional; it is normal to experience a decline in your mental health regardless of which culture you belong to and whether you have family support. Postpartum recovery involves adjusting to a major life change; thus, your struggles are real and valid. I hope by reading this section, you are able to understand yourself better from a mental health perspective.

If you or your partner are experiencing a postpartum mood disturbance, I encourage you to address and manage it together as a couple, not only to support the partner who is suffering but also to improve and strengthen your relationship. If left untreated, a prolonged mood disturbance can manifest itself in ways that can not only harm the mother's health but also harm the couple's relationship. The following are four ways in which I have commonly observed the negative impact of a postpartum mood disturbance on a couple's relationship:

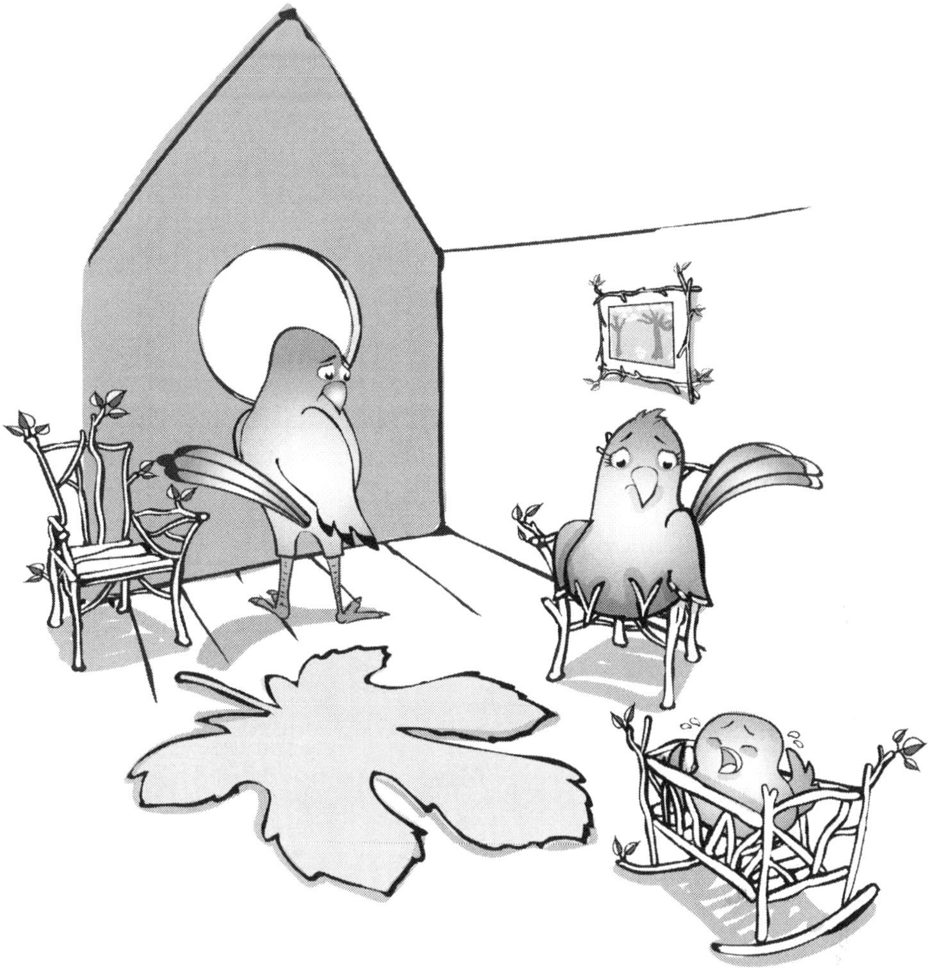

1. Mother is finding it challenging to care for herself and her baby, look after household duties, and meet her partner's needs. Her partner struggles to understand her diminishing mental health. This creates misunderstandings and feelings of resentment in both partners.

2. Mother is struggling to regulate her emotions in times of stress. With the inability to manage her emotions effectively, it reduces her capacity to communicate with her partner. This leads to increased negative interactions as her partner finds it difficult to cope and may also experience emotional dysregulation.

3. Mother is unable to effectively communicate what she needs to improve her mental health, hence, her partner is unable to adequately meet her needs. Due to unmet needs, the mother feels unsupported by her partner, making it challenging for her to meet her partner's needs. Thus, both people feel unfulfilled in the relationship.

4. Without understanding and support, the mother begins to feel disconnected from her partner. Her partner also begins to feel disconnected as they both fail to understand each other and feel confused, helpless, and/or unappreciated.

How to Improve Postpartum Mood

You may have heard of Abraham Harold Maslow, a psychologist famously known for introducing the "hierarchy of needs," which was based on his theory of human motivation (1943). Maslow argued that an individual must ensure a number of their innate needs are met in order of priority to reach their ultimate potential, or *self-actualization*. In Maslow's words, self-actualization is "the desire to become more and more what one is, to become everything that one is capable of becoming." As shown in Figure 2, he identified physiological needs as the first order of priority towards becoming your ideal self.

Based on Maslow's theory, I propose that one way you can improve postpartum mood and move a step closer to optimal health is by assessing whether your physiological needs are being met. Physiological needs are fundamental to your survival, such as food, water, air, shelter, and sleep. Unfortunately, due to the frequent demands of motherhood, women often neglect their own basic needs for survival. This includes:

- Rest
- Food
- Sleep

- Hygiene
- Exercise

Figure 2

Maslow's hierarchy of needs

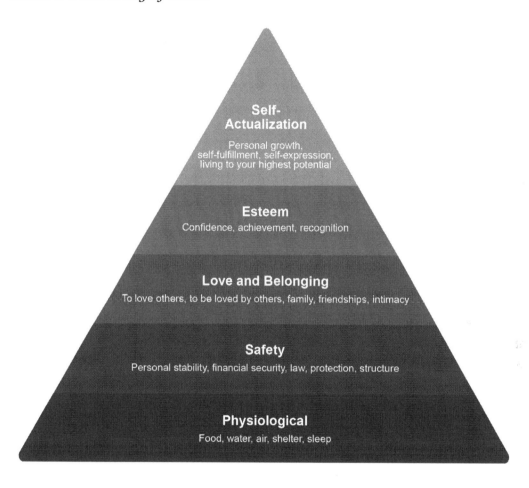
Self-
Actualization
Personal growth,
self-fulfillment, self-expression,
living to your highest potential
Esteem
Confidence, achievement, recognition
Love and Belonging
To love others, to be loved by others, family, friendships, intimacy
Safety
Personal stability, financial security, law, protection, structure
Physiological
Food, water, air, shelter, sleep

Note: Original art & material by Zara Arshad, adapted from Maslow's Hierarchy of Needs (1943)

With unmet physiological needs, mothers naturally struggle to meet their other higher order needs, such as safety and stability, belongingness, self-esteem, and self-actualization. This can lead to poor mental health and subsequent postpartum mood disturbances.

As a mother of two small children, I am also guilty of neglecting my basic human needs. Between running my mental health practice, raising two children, household duties, maintaining relationships, and meeting other demands of life, I am not very good at meeting my need for adequate sleep or nutrition. Food is an afterthought for me on most days of the week. And more than anything, I have a habit of depriving myself of enough sleep simply because I tend to procrastinate going to bed at night.

I am not alone in my habit, however. I believe sleep procrastination is a phenomenon among many mothers where they put off going to sleep to engage in activities they normally don't have time to enjoy during the day. My theory is it's common among mothers because mothers are usually the parent involved most in childcare. It is the only time of day they get to exercise their free will and think about themselves after a long day of caring for everyone else. This is also the time for mothers to connect with their partners and engage in adult conversations—uninterrupted!

However, denying your basic need for adequate sleep can result in a negative cycle of sleep deprivation, exhaustion, crankiness, irritability, unhealthy eating habits, low energy, lack of exercise, emotional dysregulation, overwhelm, inability to manage children and their needs effectively, mom guilt, and relationship distress. These factors can increase your chances of developing postpartum depression and/or postpartum anxiety.

To prevent or improve a postpartum mood disturbance, it is imperative for mothers (and fathers) to assess their sleep patterns and create change where possible. While this means you might need to reduce the number of hours of free will you enjoy at night, it does not mean you can no longer have time to yourself. You can get creative!

Here are 10 ideas for you to consider implementing to help you secure some carefree time to yourself, and hopefully motivate you to sleep earlier at night:

1. Find pockets of time during the day, such as when your baby naps.
2. Enlist your partner's help to take over baby duties for an hour at a certain time every day.
3. Wake up an hour before your baby wakes up to start your day before them.
4. If your baby goes back to sleep after an early morning feed (e.g., 4:00 a.m. or 5:00 a.m.), you can start your day instead of returning to sleep with them.
5. If you have more than one child, coordinate their nap times or quiet times to be at the same time so you can get at least an hour to yourself.
6. Use community resources, such as circle time for children at the local library, a play gym, or the sand pit at your neighborhood park where your baby will be busy and safe at the same time, allowing you to sit back and let your mind wander for a few minutes.
7. Ask for help from family members or friends during the week.
8. Go out for a walk or a car ride (that is, if your baby enjoys being in the car) and use it as your time to enjoy some peace, quiet, and coffee, as your baby looks around or naps.
9. If feasible, consider hiring a part-time nanny or a babysitter.
10. Instead of chasing time for yourself every day of the week, consider shifting your focus to creating one longer stretch of time for yourself on one or two days of the week. Perhaps on weekends, enlist the support of your partner, family member, friend, or a babysitter.

It might also be helpful to remind yourself that the phase you are in right now is a temporary one; it is limited and will pass as your baby grows. Sometimes, when you cannot do much to change your situation, it can be helpful to change your perspective towards it. Since shifting my perspective and accepting the phase of life I am in as a parent to small children, I am less inclined to chase the idea of having free will and free time in my days. I remind myself I will get to enjoy this type of freedom once again as my children grow older and need me less.

In fact, my husband and I now make a conscious effort to look for things in our days to enjoy and cherish, despite the daily chaos of life with toddlers! On particularly tough parenting days, we remind each other how this time is temporary. This makes it easier for us to approach our days with a different mindset, feel more gratitude, and develop more patience. We have not mastered this yet, but it is something we are working on together as a couple, as co-parents, and as teammates.

As you work on developing good sleep habits, remember to fulfill your other physiological needs as well. For example, allow yourself moments of rest throughout each day, especially if you did not receive adequate sleep the night before. Five to ten minutes of rest can help re-energize your body and refresh your mind, improving your overall functioning. Eating frequent nutritious meals is equally important. Consider meal planning, enlisting help from your partner or a family member, signing up for a meal service, or finding someone in your community who offers a service of fresh, home-cooked meals.

Finally, make a conscious effort to engage in physical movement. Not the kind where you are caring for your baby but the kind that improves your physical health. Once again, get creative! Attempt different ways of incorporating cardiovascular or strength training activities with your baby. For example, walk up and down the stairs a few times while wearing your baby in a carrier, put on some music and dance with your baby, do a few sets of squats or lunges as you cook dinner, or go out for a brisk walk with your baby in the stroller. Exercise is empirically validated as a natural medicine effective for reducing symptoms of depression (Cooney et al., 2013) and anxiety (Jayakody et al., 2013).

While I have suggested practical ideas to help you meet your physiological needs, I also understand it might be overwhelming for you to think about adding more things on your plate. I recognize it is not easy. I also recognize how necessary it is for you to meet your fundamental human needs to maintain and improve postpartum mental health.

As you learn to care for your child, also learn to care for yourself as a parent. Prioritizing your physiological needs by making small efforts daily is better than letting them fall to the wayside completely. Start with one need at a time, for example, adequate nutrition, and do your best to fulfill this need every day. When you are in good physical health, you are able to provide better care for your baby.

Once you determine where changes need to be made to better address your physiological needs, make a commitment to yourself and honor it with consistency and determination. From my professional experience, when mothers meet their physiological needs consistently, symptoms of postpartum depression and anxiety tend to reduce in frequency and severity. This results in a ripple effect, positively impacting overall mood, thoughts, feelings, behaviors, and the ability to cope better with external stressors, including relationship distress. I provide more information and guidance on self-care strategies in Chapter 5.

While fulfilling your physiological needs can begin to alleviate symptoms of a postpartum mood disturbance, sometimes it is not enough on its own to sustain the improvements. I believe emotional needs are as important to prioritize as your physical needs in order to maintain good mental health. In the next chapter, I explain emotional needs and how they can be adequately fulfilled.

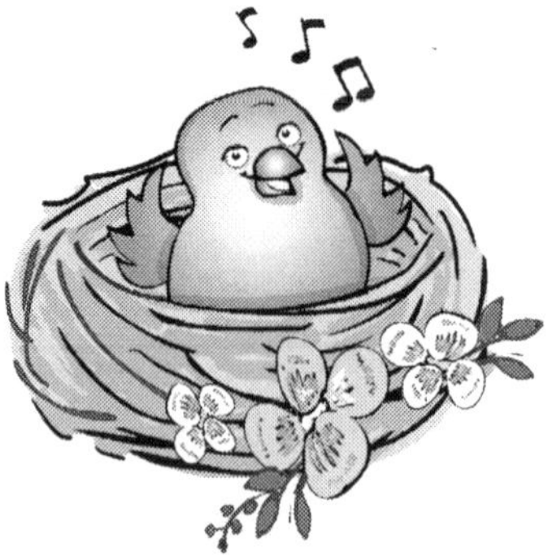

Reflections

What resonated for you in this chapter?

What are the key points you want to remember?

What might be worth discussing with your partner?

What tool or strategy do you want to put into practice?

Chapter 2: *Attachment Styles and Emotional Needs*

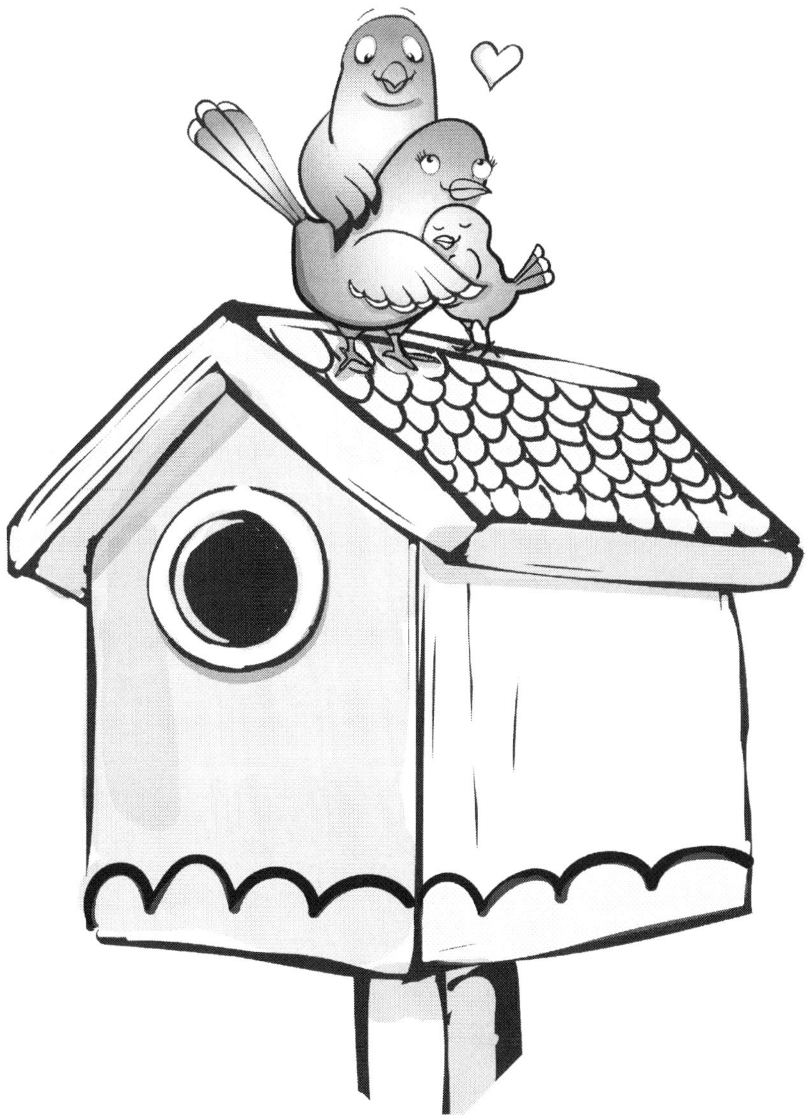

Attachment Theory

Humans are born with physical and emotional needs. While physical needs cater to our survival, such as food, water, and sleep, emotional needs provide meaning to our sense of self. Emotional needs are best understood in the context of attachment styles.

Attachment styles, as founded and developed by psychologists John Bowlby and Mary Ainsworth (Bowlby et al., 1956), form in the infancy stage, within the first 18 months of life. Based on Bowlby's theory of attachment (Bowlby, 1958), babies and young children have inherent needs to feel safe, secure, and loved. They rely on their primary attachment figures, usually their mother, father, or other primary caregiver, for their physical and emotional needs to be met.

When these needs are sufficiently fulfilled, children develop a secure attachment style. They view themselves as being safe, worthy, important, and loved and view others as safe, secure, and trustworthy. When their needs are not sufficiently fulfilled, children develop insecure attachment styles where they perceive themselves as being unsafe, unworthy, unimportant, or unloved while perceiving others as being unsafe, unstable, and unreliable to be around.

Essentially, how a parent responds to their child's needs, that is, their patterns of behavior towards the child, determines what the child comes to believe about their own self-worth and influences their perceptions of the world around them from a young age:

- *Is it safe to be with another person?*
- *Can I trust people?*
- *Am I worthy of love?*
- *Do my needs matter?*
- *Am I rejected or abandoned?*

- *Can I be close to someone?*
- *Does it feel safe to express myself openly?*
- *If no one responds to me, should I stop expressing my needs?*
- *Can I depend on others reliably?*

Depending on how a parent responds to a child's physical and emotional needs, children display one of the following attachment styles:

1. Secure
2. Anxious
3. Avoidant
4. Anxious-Avoidant (also known as Disorganized)

These four are the same attachment styles which children tend to carry forward into adulthood. As shown in Figure 3, each style of attachment can be identified by a set of characteristics that are common among people who display that particular attachment style in their adult relationships.

Figure 3

Characteristics of adult attachment styles

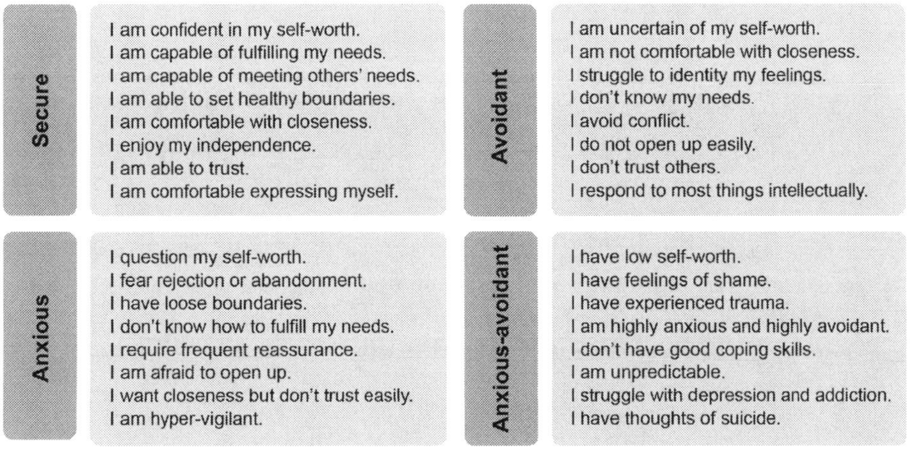
Secure
I am confident in my self-worth.
I am capable of fulfilling my needs.
I am capable of meeting others' needs.
I am able to set healthy boundaries.
I am comfortable with closeness.
I enjoy my independence.
I am able to trust.
I am comfortable expressing myself.
Avoidant
I am uncertain of my self-worth.
I am not comfortable with closeness.
I struggle to identity my feelings.
I don't know my needs.
I avoid conflict.
I do not open up easily.
I don't trust others.
I respond to most things intellectually.
Anxious
I question my self-worth.
I fear rejection or abandonment.
I have loose boundaries.
I don't know how to fulfill my needs.
I require frequent reassurance.
I am afraid to open up.
I want closeness but don't trust easily.
I am hyper-vigilant.
Anxious-avoidant
I have low self-worth.
I have feelings of shame.
I have experienced trauma.
I am highly anxious and highly avoidant.
I don't have good coping skills.
I am unpredictable.
I struggle with depression and addiction.
I have thoughts of suicide.

Let's look at this more closely as we walk through the following couple's story:

Frank and Alexis came to see me for couple's therapy because of increased tension between them. They were married and had two children together, a daughter who was three years old and a son who was 11 months old. The couple shared how Frank has a tendency to lose his temper with their children and how Alexis feels angry towards him for not listening to her and not appreciating her. I met with Alexis individually for a session to learn more about her.

From a young age, Alexis heard her parents make comparisons between her and her sister, who was two years younger. In one session, Alexis explained to me how she doesn't remember her parents ever being harsh or uncaring towards her; still, she grew up feeling she came second to her sister. She shared memories of her parents passing direct or indirect remarks comparing their two children within Alexis's earshot. She also remembered noticing differences between how her parents would treat her and her sister. For example, she remembered getting into trouble often as a child and being sent to her room as punishment, even when she didn't do anything wrong. On the other hand, her sister would get away with things easily without consequences.

Over the years, young Alexis came to believe she was not good enough because somehow, her sister was always smarter, funnier, prettier, and better in her parents' eyes. When I asked Alexis how she coped with this painful belief as a child, she shared memories of trying to gain her parents' approval in order to feel like she was enough, to feel she was as loved as her sister. Approval became Alexis's emotional need as a child.

In order to gain her parents' approval, she would try to be as obedient as possible, cleaning up after herself, trying to be the best in every sport, and studying hard to get good grades. Unfortunately, Alexis continued to feel as though she came second to her sister because her sister always received more praise and approval than she did. When she did not get the approval she so desperately needed to feel as worthy as her sister, it reaffirmed Alexis's belief that she was, in fact, not good enough. As a result of this belief, she also developed a fear of being rejected, which further fueled her need for approval. With the approval-seeking behaviors, Alexis developed skills in attuning to her parents' needs and doing things to make them happy as a way to cope with her fear of rejection.

Alexis's story demonstrates the development of an anxious attachment style. In the absence of more secure experiences in later relationships in her life, her childhood belief, *I am not good enough*, remained unchallenged. She continued patterns of high achievement, perfectionism, and people-pleasing as attempts to gain approval and fulfill her emotional need. Alexis carried these patterns into her marriage as well. She needed her husband's approval to cope with her insecure sense of worth. However, Frank was unable to meet her needs adequately as he was struggling himself. As a result of his own challenges, he did not manage his temper, nor was he able to listen to Alexis in order to understand and appreciate her more. Hence, Alexis remained anxiously attached to Frank.

While this is an example of an insecurely attached adult who has unmet emotional needs, secure children who grow into securely attached adults also have emotional needs for continued safety, security, connection, and trust. However, unlike insecurely attached adults, their innate desire to fulfill their emotional needs is not fueled by fears stemming from insecure beliefs about their worth. Rather, their desire to fulfill their needs stems from the belief that they are worthy enough to have fulfilled needs. Securely attached adults are also more likely to be proactive in meeting their own needs in healthy ways instead of solely relying on their partners.

It is important to highlight that attachment styles are not permanent. As a result of the ongoing life experiences and relationships one has, a person with a secure attachment style can develop an insecure attachment style, and vice versa. For example, a securely attached person can evolve into an insecurely attached person if they repeatedly experience a lack of safety, trust, and stability through experiences in their life. This includes abusive relationships, incessant workplace harassment, bullying, sexual trauma, discrimination, infertility, multiple losses, infidelity, loss of motor functioning due to injury, prolonged medical issues, and other such difficult experiences. On the other hand, an insecurely attached person can grow into a more securely attached person through consistent positive experiences of safety, trust, reliability, and connection, which affirm their sense of worth.

If you are in a relationship where you recognize unhealthy patterns of relating to and interacting with each other, it would be a good idea to consider seeking help from a therapist who is trained in helping couples develop secure attachments. If you are not sure about which attachment style you and your partner have, the next section will bring more clarity and help you determine your attachment style.

Identifying Your Attachment Style

If you are struggling to identify your attachment style, it might help you to know the most common type of relationship I observe among couples I support in therapy is the anxious-avoidant partnership. Sometimes, people display behaviors in both of these attachment styles, leaving them feeling confused about their attachment tendency. The best way to discover your attachment style is to identify your core beliefs and fears.

Core beliefs relate to your sense of worth, and core fears arise from the type of beliefs you hold about yourself. For example, if you believe you are unworthy, you may fear rejection. Furthermore, the type of fears you develop influence how you interpret other people's interactions with you. As demonstrated in Figure 4, your perceptions influence how you think, how you feel, and ultimately, how you behave (Beck, 2020).

Figure 4

Core factors of the anxious and the avoidant attachment styles

	Anxious Attachment	Avoidant Attachment
Beliefs	I am not good enough. I don't matter. I am unloveable. I am unworthy.	I am a failure. I am inherently wrong. I am not capable.
Fears	I will be rejected. I will be alone. I will be abandoned. People will judge me.	I will be seen as a failure. I will not succeed. I won't ever get it right.
Thoughts	I have insecure thoughts questioning my self-worth and wonder how others perceive me.	I have negative thoughts questioning my capabilities and self-worth.
Feelings	When my fears or beliefs are triggered, I feel worried, anxious, and/or stressed.	When my fears or beliefs are triggered, I feel scared, helpless, overwhelmed, and/or numb.
Behaviors	I am hyper-vigilant of my partner's reactions and needs. I engage in people-pleasing and validation-seeking behaviors. When triggered, I can become critical and attack my partner.	I am unaware of my feelings or my needs. I engage in problem-solving and success-seeking behaviors. When triggered, I can withdraw or shut down in my relationship.

When identifying your attachment style, it has less to do with how you behave and more to do with what you believe about yourself and your fears. You likely have an anxious attachment style if you can readily relate to beliefs of inadequacy or insignificance and fears of rejection, abandonment, or being judged by others, even if you display avoidant behaviors. You likely have an avoidant attachment style if you can readily relate to beliefs of being a failure and fears of not succeeding or being perceived as a failure, even if you display anxious behaviors. Let's explore this further.

Dante was 43 years old at the time he came to me for help with his feelings of depression, which he attributed to his stagnant career and conflict in his relationship. In the first session, he expressed thoughts, such as,

> *"There is no point in trying."*
> *"What will I achieve?"*
> *"It's too big to think about."*
> *"It is impossible."*

Noting a pattern in his thoughts which paralyzed him from moving forward towards his dream of achieving a successful career and his complaints about his relationship, I spent the next few sessions helping him discover his core beliefs and his attachment style:

Dante grew up in a traditional Italian family where he was the eldest of three boys and was taught from a young age to lead his siblings by setting a good example. Dante explained that in his culture, traditionally, men are expected to be strong leaders for their families. Therefore, Dante was taught to suppress his emotions and "be strong" as a child.

Dante described his father as a very angry person who was quick to lose his temper. He recalled his father yelling at him most of his childhood. He described feelings of terror and the need to cry but knowing he couldn't because it would further incite his father's anger. Instead, Dante would stand frozen in fear as his dad yelled at him, berating him for reasons he would not always understand. He would hold his tears until his father would leave and allow himself to cry when his mother would eventually come to comfort him.

As a child, Dante came to the conclusion he was not capable of achieving anything that would make his father proud of him; therefore, he developed a core belief that he is a failure. Over time, Dante became a high achiever, driven by his need to succeed in order to cope with his insecure beliefs. However, being a high achiever and fearing failure at the same time, Dante developed anxiety in his youth due to the self-imposed pressure to be the best in everything. Unfortunately, the more anxiety Dante experienced, the more he would fear failing. And the more he feared failure, the more he believed he was inherently incapable of succeeding.

As an adult, Dante became driven to have a successful career. Subconsciously, he believed that having a good career would not only make him a strong leader as a man but it would also mean he is a capable, successful person. His focus on his career created tension in his common-law relationship. After years of conflict, Dante described waking up one morning and not being able to get out of bed, like he was paralyzed. He felt heavy with a sense of doom. This was the start of Dante's battle with depression.

It took Dante several sessions to understand himself better, which came as no surprise since he had spent decades of his life suppressing himself in order to be "strong." This was also one of the reasons for conflict in his relationship. Dante shared how his partner often complained about him not having feelings nor caring about her feelings. Dante explained how he would freeze in front of his partner when she would express anger towards him, similar to his experiences in childhood. Unfortunately, this would make her angrier because she thought he didn't care about her feelings.

Dante's learned habit of suppressing his feelings and his needs, lack of insight about himself, inability to identify and name emotions, tendency to shut down in front of his partner, inability to understand his partner's feelings or needs, his fears of failure, and his need for high achievement and success all pointed to Dante having an avoidant attachment style.

Dante developed this attachment style in childhood due to unmet emotional needs; growing up, he didn't feel safe or secure in his relationships with his primary attachment figures—his parents. However, this does not necessarily mean Dante will forever remain insecurely attached in his adult relationship. With the help of his partner, it is possible for Dante to move towards secure attachment.

Developing Secure Attachment

A healthy relationship is defined by the amount of safety, security, and trust experienced in a partnership. When you and your partner are able to meet each other's physical and emotional needs, while also remaining proactive in meeting your own needs independently, it develops the safety, security, and trust in your relationship. However, these feelings do not develop in a moment. Rather, they are built in a series of moments which occur consistently over a period of time. With consistent and reliable efforts to meet each other's needs, you and your partner can grow together to form a more securely attached bond.

I emphasize consistency because without it, you cannot learn to trust each other, feel safe with one another, or maintain a strong connection in your relationship. When I say consistency, I do not mean you and your partner have to meet each other's needs *all* the time. That would be an unreasonable expectation of anyone. Instead, what I mean is you must meet each other's needs reliably *most* of the time in order to build trust and safety in your relationship.

To help the couples I work with develop secure attachments, I teach them not only to address physical and emotional needs but also to help one another develop more secure belief systems. It is vital to understand how partners in a relationship are separate individuals with distinct life experiences. For this reason, it is common for two people to have unique core beliefs, or wounds, which give birth to different emotional needs.

However, most couples who walk into my office lack fundamental insights about their partner and their individual self. Here is what I observe among these couples:

- They lack insight about each other's wounds and emotional needs.
- They lack insight about their own wounds and emotional needs.
- They trigger each other's wounds, albeit without conscious awareness.
- They are stuck in patterns of triggered wounds and unmet needs.

I will share an example of a couple, Leah and Michael, who displayed these characteristics in their partnership. This couple came to see me a few months before their marriage, when their daughter was about six weeks old. With their wedding date fast approaching, they wanted my help to improve their relationship. At the time they came to me, Leah and Michael were not very insightful or self-aware. While they knew facts about themselves and about each other, they lacked the ability to make connections between experiences in their lives, their patterns of thinking, feeling, believing, and perceiving, and how and why these patterns were showing up in their relationship. Here is what I learned about the couple as I helped them get to know themselves and understand each other better:

Michael had proposed to his girlfriend Leah about six months ago, and they recently found out they were expecting. They were both so excited! After a long battle with infertility, tired of feeling inadequate, and worrying he would leave her one day, Leah finally felt capable, confident, and happy in her relationship with Michael. On the other hand, Michael, who always felt unwanted by Leah, finally felt he was no longer disappointing her and that she was happy with him. This made it easier for Michael to be more involved with Leah and their expected baby. When the time came and their daughter was born, they were both over the moon with joy—and also very overwhelmed.

Their daughter cried every day and every night when it came time to feed. Leah could not figure out how to breastfeed her daughter. With repeated failed attempts at getting their daughter to latch on, Leah started to feel inadequate once again. The more she struggled to breastfeed and the more her daughter cried, her feelings of inadequacy grew.

Each time Michael suggested giving their daughter a bottle instead of breastfeeding, Leah interpreted his suggestion to mean that he also believed she was inadequate. She felt alone and scared. As a result, she would become angry with Michael and lash out at him. The more she lashed out, the more he believed he was disappointing her and she didn't want him around. Feeling hurt and unwanted, he would withdraw and shut himself away from her. As he became less available to her for support, Leah began to feel more alone and scared.

What Michael didn't know is that Leah yearned for his support, encouragement, and validation as her feelings of inadequacy and loneliness grew. She needed to hear from him she was a good mother, she was capable, and she was adequate despite her inability to breastfeed their daughter. She wanted to know he was there to support her through this difficult journey instead of offering quick solutions.

Michael struggled to recognize Leah's emotional needs as his own need for appreciation grew each time Leah would lash out at him. What Leah did not know is how much Michael wanted to be there for her. She didn't know how helpless he felt watching her struggle to feed their daughter every day.

In our sessions, the couple learned how Leah displayed an anxious attachment style and Michael displayed an avoidant attachment style. Both partners realized they were struggling for different reasons in the relationship. As a result of their insecure attachment styles and the stressors they were experiencing navigating parenthood, they had unique emotional needs. Leah needed Michael's validation and emotional support to feel adequate and to help soothe her anxiety. Michael needed Leah's appreciation to feel wanted and help him maintain his connection with his fiancé.

Unfortunately, both partners were unable to articulate what their needs were, therefore, neither of them knew how to help the other. Additionally, both partners were unintentionally triggering each other's wounded parts. Michael was triggering Leah's feelings of inadequacy while Leah was triggering Michael's feelings of unwantedness. As a result, they both found themselves stuck in a cycle of attack and shutdown. Both partners felt alone and misunderstood.

Based on the issues they described, it was clear to me their insecure attachment to each other was a core reason behind the couple's issues. Thus, I guided the couple towards learning how to build a more secure attachment by helping them to:

1. Discover their attachment styles
2. Articulate and understand their past and present wounds
3. Identify and describe their needs
4. Learn how to communicate their needs effectively
5. Find sustainable ways to balance both partner's needs and fulfill them consistently

By the 12th and final session, the couple reported finding it easier to implement what they were learning in therapy, despite ongoing challenges in feeding their baby. They found ways that worked well for them in gently reminding each other what their needs were when either of them was feeling triggered. Most importantly, with gentle reminders from one another, they were able to meet each other's needs consistently in the weeks leading up to the final session.

While Leah and Michael were not securely attached by the end of therapy, they were closer to developing a secure attachment than they had been at the start of therapy. The couple was laying down building blocks of a secure foundation by being mindful and responsive to each person's physical and emotional needs. Each partner was starting to trust the other more, which allowed them to be more vulnerable and gentler with each other instead of harsh or disconnected. With a vulnerable, gentle, and more connected approach in their interactions, the couple felt more safe and secure in their partnership.

As was the case between Leah and Michael, it is my observation with the couples I support that they often fail to communicate their needs to each other and are also unaware of what their own needs are. This makes me wonder, *How can anyone expect their partner to know what is needed when they don't know their own needs?* Let's take a look at the next section to learn how to identify your needs and how to communicate them to your partner.

Identifying Emotional Needs

In order to identify your emotional needs, it can be helpful to first identify your emotional wounds. Simply put, needs come from your wounds which, as demonstrated by Leah and Michael's story, can be triggered unintentionally by your partner. As a reminder, wounds, or core beliefs, often develop as a result of early childhood experiences. To help you identify your wounds, you can think about what you fear most in your relationship. Another way to discover your wound is by recognizing patterns of interactions in your relationship and uncovering the underlying reasons that fuel those patterns.

When a couple comes to see me for therapy, I closely track their patterns of behaviors by mapping out their interactional cycle. This is an effective technique developed by Sue Johnson, a prominent psychologist in the field of marriage and family therapy. When I help couples map out their interactional cycle, it helps them discover and understand how they trigger each other's wounds. Here is a list of common wounds I uncover among couples in therapy:

I am alone	I am unwanted
I am not good enough	I am unloveable
I am not worthy	I am a failure
I am not seen	I am not important
I am not heard	I don't matter
I am powerless	I am not safe

More often than not, these wounds develop during formative years in early childhood relationships with primary attachment figures—that is, parents. While most parents have no intention of harming their children, there are some parents who are intentionally abusive, whether physically, verbally, emotionally, sexually, or neglectfully. Other times, these wounds can develop in later years in unhealthy relationships. Relationships that can be damaging to one's mental health can be shared between two friends, student and teacher, manager and employee, romantically involved partners, business partners, and so on. Other times, wounds can develop as a result of traumatic experiences, such as being a target of bullying, infertility, discrimination, long-term physical injury, sexual abuse, and body shaming. Finally, these wounds can also develop in the present-day couple's relationship.

Regardless of when or how these wounds developed, couples get stuck in negative cycles caused by triggered wounds. Imagine two partners unknowingly triggering each other's wounds while reacting to each of their own triggered wounds all at the same time without conscious awareness. That is typically the process I notice among couples in therapy. Couples begin to drift apart due to angry and hurt feelings because of these triggered wounds. Hopelessness and ambivalence settle in as a result.

Once you are able to identify your emotional wound(s), think about what will provide healing. In other words, think about the opposite of the wound. If your wound is feeling inadequate, your emotional need may be to feel adequate. This emotional need can be met by your partner if you clearly communicate and request your need, making sure to clarify what type of things your partner can say or do that will help you feel adequate. Your partner is not a mind reader. They will not know what you need—or how you need it—unless you articulate it to them. Additionally, you may not have the tools to know how to communicate your needs. If this is the case, my hope is that what you are learning by reading this material will help you grow these skills.

In no particular order, here is a list of common emotional needs couples express to me in therapy:

I need acknowledgement	I need safety
I need appreciation	I need stability
I need commitment	I need respect
I need connection	I need to feel capable
I need to belong	I need to feel valuable
I need to know I matter	I need to feel seen
I need support	I need to feel heard

Another way to become aware of what your needs are is by exploring what is underneath the way you react to your partner when you are feeling triggered. For example, if you tend to become angry at your partner, what is underneath your anger?

Anger is one of the most common secondary emotions that shows up in interactions between two partners. In other words, anger is almost always a reaction to another feeling—a primary emotion (as depicted in Figure 5). That means, if you dig deeper to understand what is fueling your anger, you will discover something more vulnerable:

- Anxiety
- Exhaustion
- Fear
- Guilt
- Hurt
- Inadequacy
- Loneliness
- Loss of control
- Mistrust
- Overwhelm
- Sadness
- Stress

...and the list can go on. Typically, these primary feelings get masked by anger because it is an easier emotion to express than sharing the pain underneath. However, it usually isn't the effective emotion to express since it hardly ever achieves the desired outcome. Anger tends to spark a defensive reaction from your partner. Instead of being able to understand your feelings or your needs (which your anger is masking), your partner will feel under attack by the display of anger and respond either by shutting down, walking away, or fighting back.

Figure 5

Depiction of underlying emotions

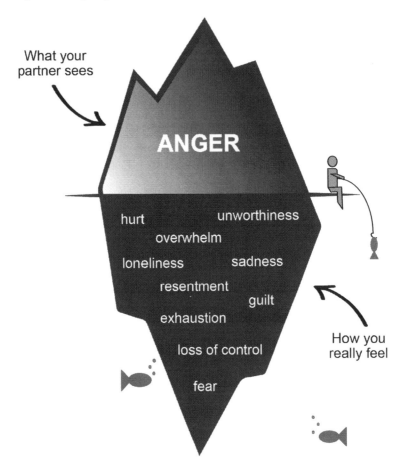
What your partner sees
ANGER
hurt
unworthiness
overwhelm
loneliness
sadness
resentment
guilt
exhaustion
loss of control
fear
How you really feel

Next time you feel angry at your partner, try to become aware of what is fueling the anger. Once you're able to identify what's underneath, try to understand it. Once you can identify and understand, evaluate what your needs are. Ask yourself, *"What need of mine is not being fulfilled at this time?"* You can refer back to page 49 to see which need(s) resonate most with you. From that place of clarity, rationality, and vulnerability, communicate with your partner. When your partner doesn't feel attacked by your anger, they will be much more likely to listen to you, understand your needs, and hopefully, respond in a helpful manner.

If you're the person usually on the receiving end of anger, and you want to help your partner articulate their needs to you, first take a moment to step back from the anger as it may be triggering for you. Stepping back can be a kind request for a time out while you gather yourself with the explicit intention of returning to the conversation. Or you can choose to remain physically present but ask for a quiet moment to check in with yourself and self-soothe. The point is to regulate your nervous system if you are feeling triggered—which is different from withdrawing or shutting down—before re-engaging in the conversation. Whatever tool you decide to use to establish or maintain emotional regulation, make sure you respectfully communicate your intention to your partner so they don't perceive you as ignoring or dismissing them. To learn about emotional regulation tools, you can read ahead to Chapter 3.

Second, once you feel more regulated, remind yourself that underneath all that anger, your partner is hurting in some way as well. Finally, respond from that place of compassion, making sure to ask questions respectfully and listen with the intent of understanding what they might be trying to tell you. If not at that moment, then later, you can say to them, *"I could see you were really angry, and I want to help. It sounds like you were saying _______. Did I understand that correctly? What can I do to help?"*

You are probably thinking, *This is easier said than done!*

I agree. It is not this easy or simple. It takes both people involved to have some level of patience, awareness, and understanding for it to be a meaningful conversation. As you embark on your journey to grow and become better partners to one another, I encourage both of you to start practicing and developing self-awareness. Learn to recognize your emotional wounds that show up when you are triggered, and become attuned to your needs. Practice emotional regulation, compassion, patience, and understanding to help you attune to your partner's needs as well, even if your partner finds it difficult to communicate their feelings to you in a helpful way. And learn to talk about these vulnerabilities with each other in a manner that brings the two of you closer together instead of drifting apart.

Xiang and Li came to me for help when their son was 16 months old. They explained how their son was born in the pandemic and how being isolated from family and friends, caring for their son, learning to be parents, and being together under the same roof had become too much for them. They described how they bickered back and forth every day over things that were not important. Over time, their bickering was turning into heated arguments. Li shared that she was quick to become angry and had a tendency to verbally attack Xiang. As I helped Li unpack her anger and understand what was underneath it, she discovered layers of resentment, feeling unseen, loneliness, and feeling unvalued.

On the other hand, Xiang expressed his frustrations around Li constantly creating more work for herself by worrying and over-planning. As I explored his frustrations further, Xiang shared how he felt rejected. When describing all the ways Li turned him down, he threw his hands in the air as he said, “She even watches all our favorite shows without me! We used to watch episodes together, but now I watch them alone at night, and she goes to bed.”

Li had tears in her eyes as she realized how rejected and hurt her husband felt. She looked down as she quietly said, “Thank you for sharing your sadness about the TV shows. I didn’t realize it upset you this much, and I will be more mindful going forward. I feel so tired and alone even though we are living under the same roof 24/7. I just want you to see me...to understand me.” Li explained how she yearned for Xiang to notice all the hard work she put into caring for their son, their house, and their family all while she was working full-time. She looked at Xiang and said, “I want you to see me and value my hard work. I know you think I am overdoing it, but it makes me angry and resentful when you dismiss whatever I’m doing as being unnecessary. What I do is important to me. And I hope you can come to understand that about me."

As the couple shifted to more softened stances towards each other, I helped them work through their interactional patterns and identify their wounds. They both seemed to carry resentment towards one another. Xiang felt resentful because he was tired of feeling rejected for the past 16 months. Li felt resentful because she felt alone, unseen, and unvalued. These wounds, as I learned through explorative work in sessions, were not new to Li or Xiang. They both were able to recognize when and how they developed these wounds in past relationships and how each of them was reliving these wounds in their present relationship with each other. Neither wanted to hurt the other, yet both were unconsciously triggering each other's wounded parts.

As we started working towards identifying emotional needs and learning to communicate them, Xiang shared, "Li, I feel rejected, and it makes me resentful towards you. I don't like feeling this way. I miss how we used to be. I know it isn't possible to have our former relationship especially since we are together all the time under the same roof with our son, but it would be nice to know you want to spend time with me. I need to feel wanted by you."

When it was Li's turn to articulate her needs, she said, "The reason I don't feel like spending time with you anymore is because I feel bitter and angry towards you. I'm angry because I feel so alone and unvalued each time you criticize or dismiss my efforts when I am trying to do my best to fulfill my duties as a mother, as a wife, and as a homemaker all while working too! It would make such a difference to me if I knew you appreciated me for all that I do."

As demonstrated by Xiang and Li's story, the couple was stuck in a negative cycle. Li's anger towards Xiang, which masked her loneliness and resentment, came in the way of her wanting to be with her husband. As a result, she would decline his efforts to connect with her. Xiang felt this rejection deeply. He resented his wife for putting so much effort into everything but him. Naturally, he became dismissive and sometimes condescending towards Li and her efforts.

With a few sessions of couple's therapy, newfound awareness developed, and the couple began meeting each other's needs with conscious effort. Instead of bickering about the dishes, the pile of laundry, whose turn it was to give their son a bath, or the toys strewn around the living room, they started communicating vulnerably and attuning to each other's needs. They expressed if they felt rejected or dismissed and gently reminded each other about what would be helpful instead.

Imagine how different your interactions can be with your partner once both of you are aware of your unhealed parts that are being triggered and your subsequent needs. Moreover, imagine the positive impact it can have on your relationship and your attachment when both of you become mindfully aware of each other's unhealed parts, learn to anticipate needs accordingly and respond to them appropriately. Wouldn't that be nice? Yet, like Xiang and Li, so many couples struggle to recognize each other's wounds and meet each other's needs.

Here are the main reasons why I believe couples lack this ability:

- Lack of insight: one or both partners don't know what their emotional needs are or what their partner's needs are
- Lack of self-awareness: one or both partners are unable to recognize their patterns or attune to their needs
- Lack of tools to support good communication
- Lack of tools to support emotional regulation
- Unreasonable or unspoken expectations

- Imbalance of needs: one partner works harder to meet the other partner's needs at the expense of their own mental health (example: pleasing behaviors, walking on eggshells, or suppressing their needs)

Building and Maintaining Emotional Connection

When emotional needs are consistently left unfulfilled, it impacts a couple's emotional connection. Emotional connection is the degree to which two people mutually share a felt sense of comfort, closeness, trust, and understanding in each other's presence. Emotional connection doesn't occur overnight. Rather, it is built over time through meaningful exchanges between two partners. It also ebbs and flows based on the varying experiences and stages of a relationship. For example, a couple might feel more connected during pregnancy and less connected after their child is born.

Therefore, not only does emotional connection need to be built in a relationship, it also has to be maintained through conscious effort. If you notice you and your partner are feeling less connected, or not connected at all, it's a good time to tune inwards and recognize which wounds are aching and what needs are unfulfilled. Once you and your partner are able to recognize your unmet needs and turn to each other for support, connection can be reestablished.

Something that contributes to harming a couple's connection instead of strengthening it is the common misunderstanding that it is your partner's responsibility to read your mind and satisfy all of your needs. While your partner is partly responsible for meeting your needs in order to establish and maintain a secure connection, they cannot be held solely responsible. Ideally, your romantic relationship serves as one of several resources you can tap into for meeting your needs.

During the times you rely on your partner for fulfilling your needs, you have to be mindful of how you communicate your expectation. If you make demands of them to satisfy your needs, they will likely feel as though they are being told what to do. In most cases, people don't react well to feeling controlled or forced into doing something. Therefore, making demands will likely break your connection with your partner. Instead, when you make a request by gently asking your partner if they would be willing to consider your needs, it allows them autonomy and conveys mutual respect. A beautiful example of this is when Li kindly requested Xiang to honor her hard work by demonstrating appreciation.

Figure 6

Different ways of fulfilling your emotional needs

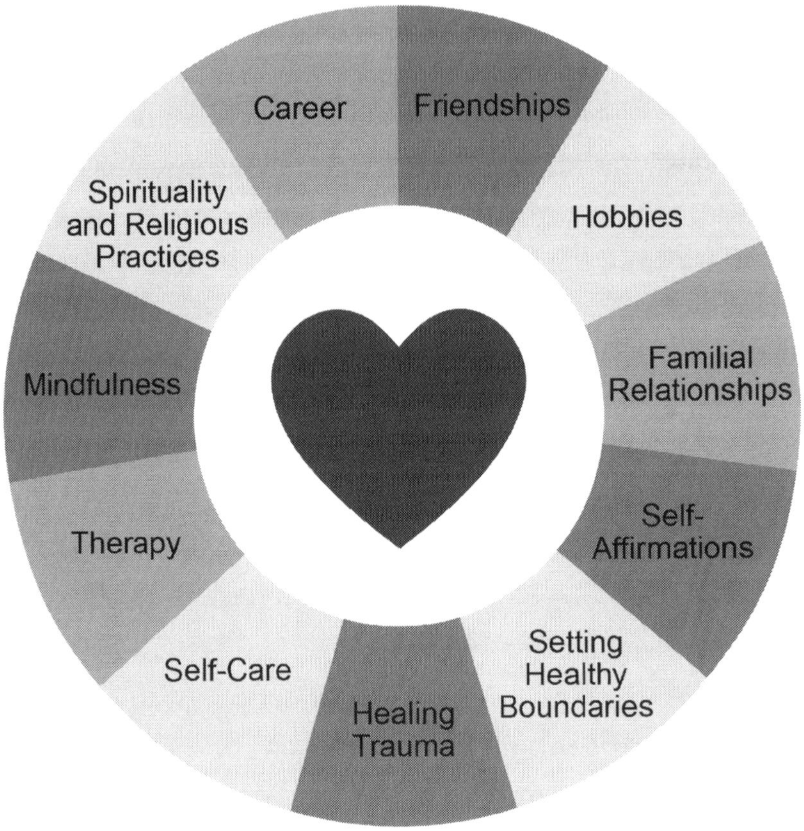
Career
Friendships
Hobbies
Familial Relationships
Self-Affirmations
Setting Healthy Boundaries
Healing Trauma
Self-Care
Therapy
Mindfulness
Spirituality and Religious Practices

While some physical and emotional needs are more specific to a romantic relationship, many are not exclusive to it. As showcased in Figure 6, emotional needs can be fulfilled in a number of ways outside of your relationship. Couples who have access to other avenues for satisfying their individual needs share a more fulfilling partnership because it takes the pressure off of one partner feeling like they must be the source of fulfillment for the other. This also maintains a healthy balance in the relationship where both individuals share mutual autonomy and mutual dependance. Striking this balance helps two people build trust and security in the relationship, which increases emotional connection.

Ruptures and Repairs

Conflict is inevitable in relationships. Disagreements, arguments, and other negative interactions occur in most relationships, even in the most secure ones. In fact, if you share a healthy, balanced partnership which encourages autonomy of the two individuals involved, I don't believe it is possible to eliminate conflict entirely. Partnerships that are void of conflict don't experience the same opportunities of deepening connection as partnerships that face conflict. Conflict presents an opportunity to create understanding, healing, growth, and ultimately, a deepened connection.

Drs. John and Julie Gottman, renowned psychologists known for their research on marital stability and predicting divorce, have studied countless couples and come to the conclusion that conflict is not the problem; rather, how it is managed and what the couple does afterwards can be problematic. The Gottmans refer to this concept as ruptures and repairs, or the breaking and restoring of connection between two people.

Are you a couple that becomes cold, distant, and silent towards each other after conflict? Or are you angry, harsh, and spiteful? These are the behaviors that can intensify and prolong hurt feelings, making the process of resolution more difficult in your relationship. On the other hand, if you are a couple who is able to turn towards each other to resolve the issue, make sincere amends, and move forward with mutual respect and understanding, then you are effectively repairing the rupture. In other words, you are rebuilding your connection.

From an attachment perspective, consistent repairs are necessary to develop and maintain a mutual sense of safety and trust in your relationship. Consistency helps you anticipate amends following a threat to your attachment bond. This contributes to building a secure attachment to one another.

When you and your partner are able to turn towards one another soon after conflict with the intention of making amends, not only does it resolve lingering feelings such as hurt or anger, it also brings you closer. Turning towards each other during a repair attempt includes:

1. Acknowledging the conflict with compassion
2. Communicating more vulnerably the second time
3. Sincerely make an effort to understand the other better
4. Owning up to one's own contribution in the negative interaction
5. Extending a sincere apology

Depending on the nature and level of severity of the conflict, a repair attempt can also be achieved nonverbally or indirectly in the following ways:

- A kiss on the forehead
- A joke to lighten the mood
- A quiet, meaningful hug
- An offer to help with something
- A suggestion to watch a movie together
- An unsolicited shoulder rub

Remember, the point of a repair attempt is to rebuild the connection. Ultimately, you are doing something to let each other know you still care for and love each other. By doing so, you are also cultivating safety and security in the relationship.

While it can be difficult to think of turning towards your partner for reconnection soon after an argument or a fight, it can be even more difficult to sit with hurt or angry feelings for a prolonged period. Which difficult road do you want to choose and for what consequence?

Without a doubt, turning towards your partner will feel challenging the first few times, but it will feel easier the more you practice it. Think of it this way: During conflict, you either walk away or become harsh out of habit. Therefore, it becomes a matter of developing a new habit to respond differently through consistent practice. You can never be in the wrong when you approach your partner with loving intentions and say, *"Hey, that didn't go so well. I don't like how I reacted, and I am sorry. Can we have a redo of the conversation and be more mindful of how we are communicating this time? I know we have the ability to resolve this and get back to a better place."*

While repairs positively influence connection, there are a few things that negatively influence it. In the following section, I will share some of the things I have come to observe in my professional experiences which serve as obstructions to establishing a strong connection.

What Inhibits Emotional Connection?

There are times when a couple finds it difficult to establish emotional connection. This can happen when there are reasons which inhibit a person's ability to meaningfully connect with their partner. Here are the common reasons I have come to discern which I will highlight in the following way:

1. **Unresolved attachment injury.** Dr. Sue Johnson describes an attachment injury as "a feeling of betrayal or abandonment during a critical time of need" (Johnson et al., 2001). In other words, when a person is emotionally unavailable, responds inadequately, or abandons their partner at a time of critical need, it can result in an injury to the couple's attachment bond. When this injury is left unresolved, a part of the wounded partner remains stuck in that period of time. This part of them continues to hurt deeply, preventing them from meaningfully connecting in the relationship.

   Attachment injuries can be caused by unchecked rage, a breach of trust, unjust accusations, gaslighting, addiction, abuse, lying, manipulating, not responding to your partner's reasonable requests during a time of need, talking negatively about your partner behind their back, having an affair, minimizing your partner's feelings, and other such harmful behaviors.

   While the injured partner may appear to be showing up as they normally would in the relationship, things may be different below the surface. Because of the unresolved pain they are carrying from the attachment injury, these individuals are no longer able to trust their partner or feel emotionally safe with them. They may also be carrying feelings of resentment, betrayal, anger, disappointment, and sadness, regardless of how much time has passed.

   Sometimes these individuals are not aware of the pain they are carrying, don't know how to articulate it to their partner and ask for what they need to heal, or their partner has not been able to respond appropriately to their request for healing. Thus, it inhibits the wounded partner's ability to connect. Additionally, the impact of the attachment injury and the lack of emotional connection can spill over into affecting the couple's physical intimacy.

In order to rebuild the trust and connection in the relationship, the injured partner usually requires a healing event or moment to take place within the relationship before they can move on from the impact of the injury. In therapy, I help the couple make sense of the attachment injury and find healing through a series of steps which involve:

- Creating space for the injured partner to narrate the event from their perspective and articulate their pain

- Encouraging the second partner to listen and remain present instead of reacting, defending, minimizing, or otherwise interrupting

- Helping the second partner in providing sufficient validation to the hurting partner, expressing their sincere remorse and explaining why their partner can trust it will not happen again

- Helping both partners identify and agree upon new behaviors the second partner needs to demonstrate consistently in order to reestablish safety in the relationship (not just words, but actions!)

- If the injured partner is open to it, I assist the second partner to narrate the event from their perspective non-defensively, helping them discover and identify underlying issues which could bring clarity to both partners and facilitate the process of healing

2. **Unresolved or ongoing trauma.** Trauma can be a single event, or a series of events, which severely dysregulates a person's nervous

system and impacts their ability to cope or feel safe. In a relationship context, these events can include:

- Abuse (emotional, verbal, physical, or sexual)
- Infidelity
- Attachment injury
- Coping with addiction
- Prolonged unmet needs

Trauma creates damage to the relationship because it can instantaneously break the connection between two people. When trauma remains unresolved, or it continues in the relationship, it shakes the foundational requirements of a healthy, securely attached partnership: trust, safety, and security. Without trust, safety, and security between two intimately involved people, it can wreak havoc on one or both partners' mental health. Not only does it prevent a traumatized partner from reaching out to the other, it can also prevent the other partner from establishing connection due to feelings of shame.

3. **Cultural norms and values.** In a previous section, I established the importance of fulfilling needs in order to build connection and secure attachment between two people. However, I have noticed that communicating needs does not come naturally in some relationships, in particular among couples with non-Western cultural backgrounds. While celebrating and honoring cultural heritage is valuable and oftentimes enjoyable, some of these cultural backgrounds support particular norms and values which I believe inhibit a couple's ability to fulfill important needs in order to meaningfully connect.

   Considering how my upbringing has been strongly influenced by South Asian culture, I would have also struggled to communicate my needs directly to my husband had it not been for my exposure to Western values and my training as a therapist. On the contrary, it has taken my husband nine years of being married to a therapist to finally come to terms with the fact that he has emotional needs as well and it is okay to express them! As the eldest born son of a South Asian family, my husband made it his duty to serve his family. To think of himself and what he needs was a selfish idea to him up until recently. And he is not alone in his thinking. To serve, to be selfless, and to maintain harmony by forgoing your own wants and needs are values strongly upheld in many Eastern cultures, both among men and women. Many religions also uphold similar values.

In my opinion, maintaining cultural and religious values is important to your sense of identity, belonging, and faith. At the same time, I also believe it is important to apply critical thinking skills to understand their place and purpose in your life and relationships. For example, in cultures where selflessness is valued, is the purpose of the value to keep people unhappy, lonely, burnt out, or unfulfilled? Or is the purpose of the value to promote compassion, empathy, responsibility, charity, strength, connection, and love in relationships?

On another note, it is also important to be mindful of what other values you are sacrificing at the expense of upholding one particular value. For example, if being selfless and maintaining harmony are two important values in your culture or religion, how harmonious is your relationship with your partner if you both are working to serve the needs of the family and forgoing your individual and relationship needs? With enough time gone by, chances are either tensions will rise or distance will occur in your relationship, leading you to disconnect from each other. Hence, your relationship may feel more resentful and discontented rather than harmonious. In this case, I'd argue it would be better for both partners to learn to balance the needs of the family with their individual and relationship needs so they can share a more fulfilled and harmonious partnership.

Finally, I believe communicating needs with your partner is not being selfish, nor is it a sign of weakness. Rather, it is an act of courage, commitment, strength, and connection. When you are communicating your needs to your partner, you are essentially saying, *"This relationship is important to me, and I want to make sure I bring the best version of myself into it. I am my best version of myself when my needs are considered and I can maintain good mental health."*

4. **Assumptions.** I frequently notice a tendency among couples to assume their partner knows what they need. Mind reading is not a power many people are born with, yet people expect their partner to read their mind and know exactly what it is they need and how to meet that need. The irony about this is many people I work with feel upset with their partner for not instinctively knowing what to do, yet these individuals are not aware of their own needs nor their partner's needs!

   Silently expecting your partner to know what to do is unfair to the relationship and can inhibit you from meaningfully connecting with one another. I address this topic further in Chapter 5. Additionally, people often make the mistake of assuming their partner's intentions behind something they did or didn't do without giving them a chance to clarify by asking directly in a non-accusatory tone. Making assumptions in this manner can be harmful to two people's connection. If you frequently engage in creating potentially inaccurate narratives in your mind about your partner, it can influence your feelings and behaviors towards them, ultimately inhibiting your ability to connect.

5. **Poor communication.** Based on my experience working with couples, one of the biggest obstructions to emotional connection is poor communication. When couples complain about unmet needs despite communicating them to their partner, I observe their interactions in therapy sessions and come to notice poor communication strategies. In these cases, it is no wonder both partners feel unheard, misunderstood, and unfulfilled. With ineffective communication and unfulfilled needs, individuals begin to feel hurt and resentful. These feelings can hold each partner back from connecting with one another.

   Helping individuals communicate effectively with their partners is a large part of the work I do in supporting postpartum couples as they navigate their relationship after baby. In the next section, I will share effective strategies and tools that you can use in your relationship to improve communication. Learning and implementing healthy communication skills will lead to a more emotionally fulfilled and securely attached relationship between you and your partner.

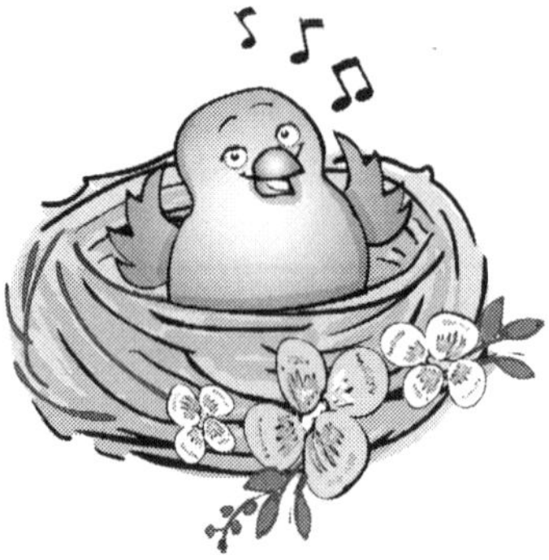

Reflections

What resonated for you in this chapter?

What are the key points you want to remember?

What might be worth discussing with your partner?

What tool or strategy do you want to put into practice?

Chapter 3: *Communication*

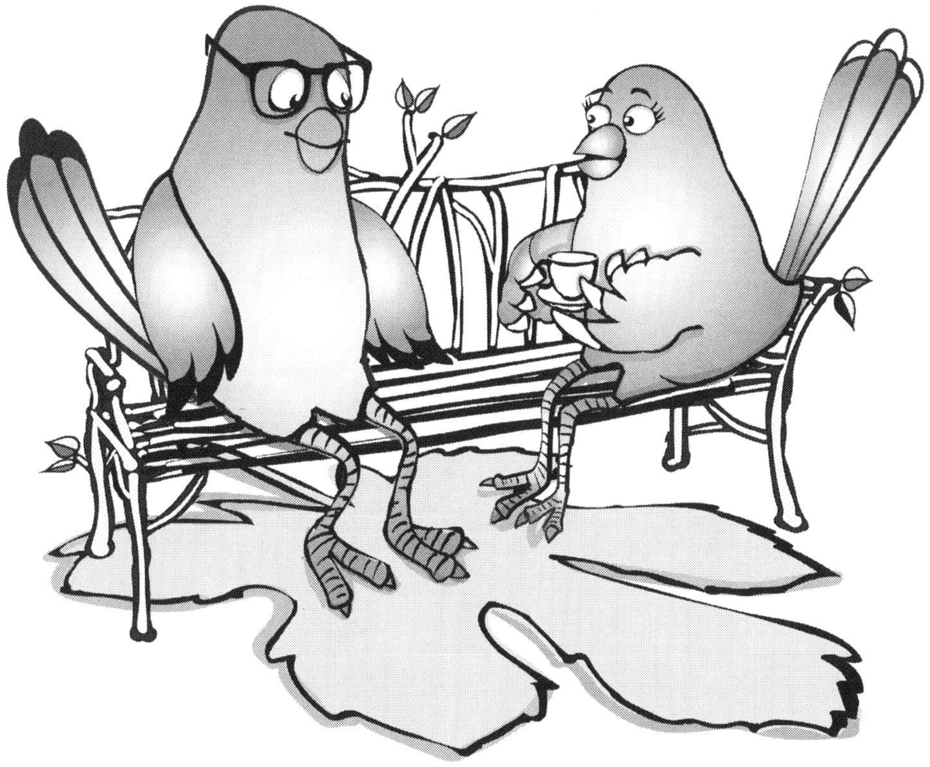

Four Common Mistakes in Communication

While there are many reasons why couples seek my services, inability to communicate is the most common reason they share in the first session.

Why is that?

Communication is not simply an exchange of words between two people. It is an interaction which is laden with subjective experiences which include thoughts, feelings, perspectives, fears, beliefs as well as tone of voice, facial expressions, and body language. Thus, when two people with unique thought patterns, emotions, perceptions, fears, and beliefs come together to form an intimate relationship, it is natural to experience challenges in talking with and understanding each other.

Difficulties in communication are more likely to arise in stressful or challenging situations, such as the time when a new baby joins the family. However, the more time passes with harmful interactions between two partners, layers of misunderstandings, hurt, anger, and other emotions are created within the relational dynamic. Overtime, the damage deepens, and communication patterns become destructive.

Let's take a look at the story of Mona and Liam, a married couple with a seven-month-old son who came to see me for 11 sessions. Liam worked full-time, and Mona was continuing her journey of pursuing higher education during her maternity leave. In the first session, the couple described reaching a point in their marriage where they no longer found it possible to resolve any issues. They described damaging communication patterns and wanted help to improve their communication so they could resolve their issues more successfully. Here is how they displayed their vicious communication cycle in one session:

Mona and Liam sat at a distance from each other on the couch, facing forward with stern expressions and only maintaining eye contact with me. They both expressed their frustrations, sharing how neither of them felt safe to reach out for emotional support from the other. Mona described feelings of depression within the first year of their marriage due to experiencing two miscarriages. According to Mona, Liam was not there for her; she felt alone in her grief as she suffered the pain of the losses. She continued on to share her experience of postpartum depression and anxiety a year later when their son, Oliver, was born. Once again, Mona described feeling alone in her suffering without any emotional support forthcoming from Liam. With a shaking voice and tears rolling down her face, she described feeling exhausted and lonely.

At first, Liam listened quietly with a hardened look on his face. Then he began interrupting her, defending himself with combative body language and hand gestures as he spoke directly to his wife. He angrily described all the ways he had been there for Mona and everything he did to share responsibilities in caring for Oliver. "I make her breakfast every morning, I make sure all the bottles are washed and dishes are cleaned, I do my best to give her breaks, and all she does is complain and accuse me of not helping her. I am sick of it!"

This time, it was Mona's turn to become quiet and hardened. Looking at me, she retorted how the weight of responsibility of feeding their son every two hours for the past seven months had fallen on her. She was angry as she explained how Liam didn't understand the toll this took on her. She repeated how exhausted she was, how she hadn't slept in months, how she had been studying for exams the past few weeks with little sleep or time to herself, and how unfair it was for Liam to head to bed early every night without a care for her. "I am trying to wean Oliver off breastfeeding, and every time I ask Liam to help me with bottle feeding, he conveniently gives up at the first sign of resistance from Oliver, hands him back to me, and goes off to sleep. How am I supposed to attend my classes or get a job if he doesn't help me with getting Oliver to start taking the bottle?! He takes me for granted and treats me like I'm some kind of a baby-feeding machine!" Mona exclaimed.

Not surprisingly, these statements were enough to set Liam off again, defending himself vehemently and shifting the blame back to her. I watched the couple argue for a few minutes, noticing how they attacked each other back and forth, blaming the other for problems in their relationship without taking a moment to really understand what the other was experiencing. Their argument ended in silence and cold, distant expressions.

Mona and Liam's communication cycle showcases several communication pitfalls which are considered a bad omen for marital stability. In his book *The Seven Principles of Making Marriage Work* (Gottman & Silver, 2000), Dr. John Gottman outlines four common communication errors among married couples who eventually divorced. These findings are based on decades' worth of research he conducted in his famous "Love Lab," a couple's laboratory he opened in 1986—the first of its kind. These communication mistakes are presented in Figure 7.

Figure 7

Four communication errors discovered by Drs. John and Julie Gottman

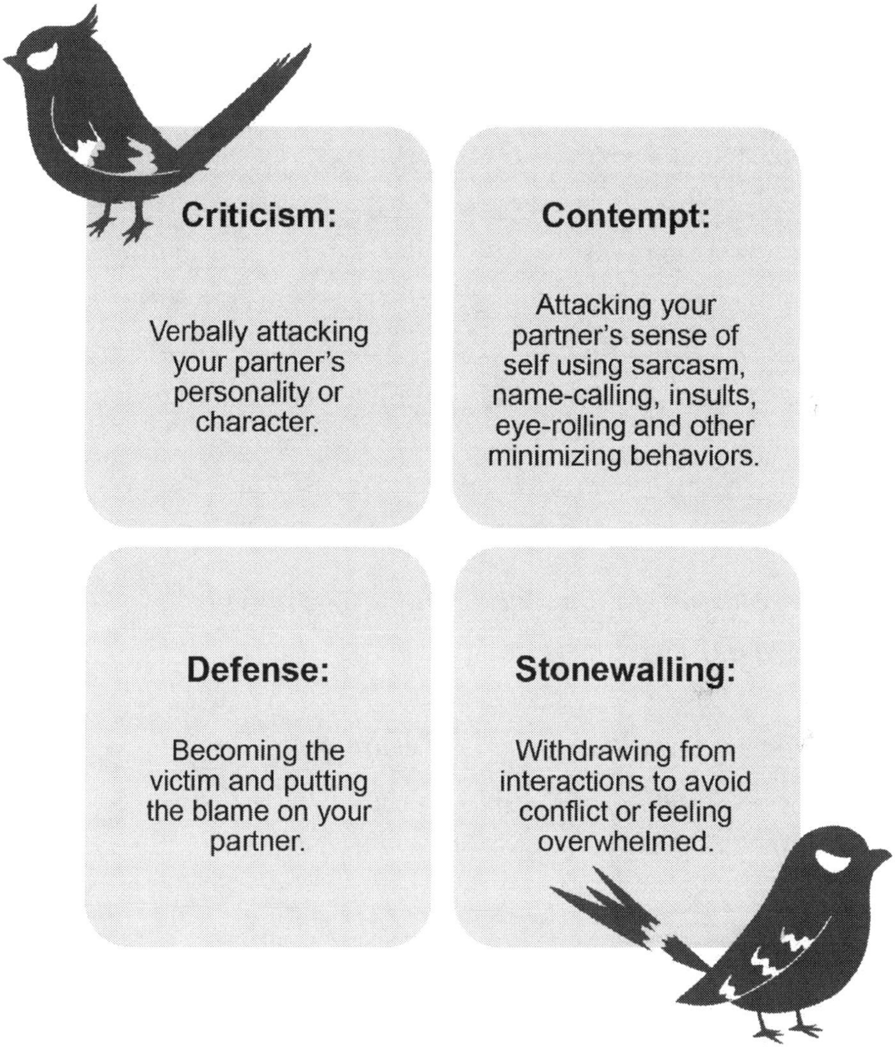
Criticism:
Verbally attacking your partner's personality or character.
Contempt:
Attacking your partner's sense of self using sarcasm, name-calling, insults, eye-rolling and other minimizing behaviors.
Defense:
Becoming the victim and putting the blame on your partner.
Stonewalling:
Withdrawing from interactions to avoid conflict or feeling overwhelmed.

Dr. Gottman discovered that spouses developed these patterns of communication over time, often without conscious awareness. He also argued that these errors don't show up at the same time in a couple's relationship; they make their way one by one as time goes on.

Furthermore, he found that the occasional presence of some of these communication errors is not what indicates divorce. Instead, it is the persistent presence of all these errors that may indicate a couple's marriage is heading for trouble.

Does that mean you will get divorced? No, but it means it's time to make some necessary changes to improve the health of your relationship. I have broken down each of these common mistakes in detail and provided suggestions which may help you and your partner in improving your communication. My hope is for you to unlearn harsh and damaging communication strategies and instead, learn to develop softer and more effective ways of communicating. By improving how you interact with each other, I believe you can have a more fulfilled, loving, and well-connected partnership.

Criticism

1. *"You're always playing video games. You don't care to spend any time with me."*

2. *"I'm sick of doing the dishes and cleaning the house when I come home tired from work. You are home all day; why can't you clean up after yourself?"*

3. *"You never listen to anything I say, so I'm done talking."*

4. *"When is the last time you initiated sex? I don't see how this will work if you don't put in any effort into our relationship."*

5. *"You are so inconsiderate! You lock yourself down in the basement every day to work, and you don't even*

bother to come up even once to ask if I need a break or help with the kids."

6. *"Why does everything have to be your way? Loosen up!"*

If any of the above statements sound familiar to you, you and/or your partner might have a tendency towards being critical of the other. As Gottman would describe them, criticisms tend to be global statements which convey a negative sentiment about a person. Anytime you catch yourself using phrases like "you always," "you never," or any other kind of absolute statement, recognize that you're pointing out a fault in your partner's character because you're indicating that if they are *always* or *never* doing something, then they must have a faulty part in their personality. Most people on the receiving end of such criticisms would agree this doesn't sit well with them.

Additionally, saying words like "always" or "never" shifts your partner's focus to defending themselves by pointing out exceptions to when they did or didn't do something. This takes away from their ability to focus on understanding what you might be trying to convey to them.

A conversation that starts with a criticism is bound to go south. This is what Gottman would refer to as a harsh start-up, which is another sign he has found to predict divorce (Gottman & Silver, 2000). In his "Love Lab" research, Gottman observed when a partner began a conversation with a criticism, an attack, or an otherwise mean comment, the conversation typically escalated towards conflict. This created angry and hurt feelings and usually led to no resolve at the end of the interaction.

This is no different than what I observe among couples in my practice. Whenever I notice one partner start a conversation with a statement that somehow puts the other partner down, it immediately sparks a reaction from the partner who is the recipient of the insult. Whether the reaction is loud and angry or silent and disengaged, the tension escalates quickly.

Some of you may be wondering by now, "How am I supposed to talk to my partner when I am feeling frustrated or upset about something?"

The answer is, try to communicate your feelings in the form of a concern versus a criticism. Why? Because a concern lands softer than a criticism. However, you should be mindful of how you are forming your concern because it can easily cross over into criticism. Gottman (Gottman & Silver, 2000) identifies three components which can help you communicate your concern most effectively:

1. A specific incident
2. Your feeling(s) about it
3. An explicit need or request

To demonstrate, let's use the six criticisms from the start of this section and turn them into concerns:

1. *"I noticed while I was waiting to spend time with you last night, you chose to play video games for two hours* **(specific incident)**. *I felt disconnected and alone* **(feeling)**. *I understand you need to decompress after a stressful day at work. Would you also be willing to set some time aside for us to be together in the evenings before we go to bed* **(explicit request)***?"*

2. *"I'm feeling frustrated right now* **(feeling)**. *I just finished cleaning up the pile of dishes in the sink and putting away the toys in the family room* **(specific incident)**. *When I come home, I am usually*

exhausted **(feeling),** *and all I want to do is relax and spend time with my family* **(need).** *Can we discuss a better way to share these responsibilities* **(explicit request)***?"*

3. *"It makes me feel like I'm not important* **(feeling)** *when I am talking to you and you are distracted by what the baby is doing* **(specific incident).** *Can you please give me your undivided attention for a few minutes* **(specific request)***? I need someone to talk to right now* **(need).** *And if now is not a good time, can you please let me know when we can talk* **(specific request)***?"*

4. *"I felt disappointed* **(feeling)** *last night when I initiated sex and you told me you were too tired and went to sleep* **(specific incident).** *I feel alone and confused* **(feeling)** *because I don't know what's happening between us. I think it's important for us to address this and figure it out together* **(need).***"*

5. *"I didn't feel this way before Arlo was born, but now it makes me resentful* **(feeling)** *when I see you lock yourself down in the basement and work all day* **(specific incident).** *I am alone caring for him, and I need your support* **(need).** *It would be so helpful if you could come upstairs during your lunch hour so I can catch a break. Is that something you'd be willing to do* **(specific request)***?"*

6. *"I feel angry* **(feeling)** *when you're raising your voice at me right now* **(specific incident).** *I understand you like things a certain way, but it's*

important for me to feel respected too **(need)**. *I need to know my voice and my way of doing things also matters in this relationship* **(need)**.*"*

In reading through these examples, your first thought may be, "Who talks like this?! This isn't realistic."

I agree that it may feel unnatural to speak in this manner likely because you are not in the habit of communicating this way. Once you make the effort to develop the habit, you will begin to communicate in a manner similar to the examples above, but in words that come more naturally to you. And the truth is, expressing a concern does not necessarily mean your conversation will not turn into an argument. It might. However, my experience working with couples is that when both partners practice communicating in the manner I presented, there are fewer opportunities for either partner to become triggered and reactive. Thus, conversations don't become as heated.

Willingness and consistent practice from both partners is key to creating long-lasting positive changes in your communication cycle. Think of it this way: If you have something to say, why not make it count by expressing yourself in a way that increases your chances of being heard and understood? It might not be easy in the beginning—it might even feel awkward or uncomfortable. Eventually, it will come more naturally to you, and hopefully become second nature to communicate this way. Give it a try!

HOW TO EXPRESS A COMPLAINT

- ✔ Focus on a specific incident or situation.
- ✔ Share what feelings came up as a result of it.
- ✔ Express a request or a need at the end.
- ✔ Use "I" statements.
- ✔ Avoid the words *always* and *never*.

Defensiveness

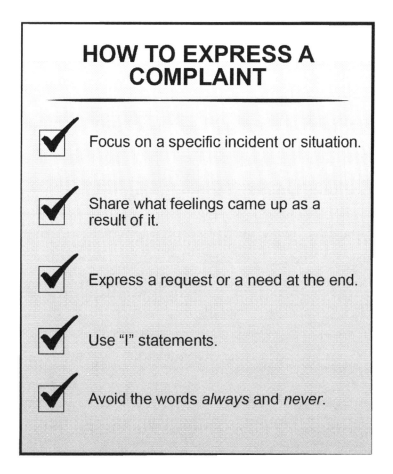

Have you ever noticed when you try to defend yourself in an argument, it does not stop your partner from continuing to blame you? That's because your partner may be feeling invalidated, or they might be hearing you say, *"The problem is not with me, it is with you!"* For some of you, defensiveness can be a way to shift the blame on to your partner and, as a result, make yourself the victim. Thus, defensiveness tends to escalate an argument rather than defuse it. Rarely will your partner back down and say, *"Okay, I'm sorry, I understand."*

Here is an example of a defensive response to an expressed concern:

Fred: *"Whenever I try to spend time with you, you often push me away. You're either working or with the kids. You don't make time for us!"*

Catherine: *"I'm exhausted by the end of the day. You don't know how tiring it gets. I just need some space and time alone. You should understand that."*

While it may be normal for Catherine to defend herself, all Fred heard was an excuse to blow him off, his complaint not being taken seriously, and feeling blamed for not being more understanding. Chances are a defensive response like Catherine's will escalate the interaction. Fred may become angry and defensive with her, or he might withdraw from the conversation despite feeling hurt.

Here are three ways you can respond when your partner brings up a concern to you:

1. **Accept responsibility.** It may be difficult to accept responsibility when you feel criticized or blamed for something. However, what is the point of defending yourself when it will only fuel the conflict further instead of making things better? Keep in mind that you have the option to explain yourself at another time after the conflict is defused.

   Consider trying something new by accepting responsibility—at least for your part in the issue—and see how things progress. Using Catherine's example, here is how she can accept responsibility:

   "Thank you for sharing and bringing this to my attention. I struggle to balance everything between kids, work, and the house. This leaves me tired by the end of the day, and I tend to forget to make time for us. I do need to work on prioritizing time for us too.

I care about your feelings, and I also appreciate you understanding how stretched thin I am right now."

2. **Be curious and listen to understand.** It is imperative to remember that your partner has needs as well. They want to be heard and understood, as much as you want them to listen and understand you. However, they might be making the mistake of expressing themselves harshly, which will likely bring out a negative reaction from you. By allowing yourself to react, you are no longer present. You are either in your head thinking of ways to respond or feeling too overwhelmed with emotion to pay attention.

   Instead, take a deep breath, stay present with yourself, then do your best to shift your stance to that of curiosity. Ask questions non-defensively with the intention of stepping in your partner's shoes for a few moments and sincerely making an effort to understand them. This is when you refrain from interrupting them and avoid rebuttals, debates, or any kind of response where you are trying to prove them wrong. What's more, when you ask questions gently, respectfully, and compassionately, it can positively influence your partner to soften their stance towards you.

   Here is an example of how Catherine can practice curiosity, allowing her an opportunity to really listen and understand Fred:

   "I get so tired juggling everything that by the end of the day, I just want to be alone. You are right, Fred, I haven't been paying attention to how this might make you feel. Can you help me understand what it's like for you when I push you away?"

   When you remain open and curious in this manner, it makes it possible for you to receive and absorb new information. Absorbing new information creates opportunities for new perspectives, learning, and growth.

3. **Consider needs and/or requests.** Another way to prevent an escalation of conflict is by recognizing your partner's needs and acknowledging them. Avoid presenting your own needs as a way to dismiss your partner's needs. Remember, this is not a competition of whose needs are more important. You are both worthy of having your needs fulfilled. Hence, if you have unmet needs, you can share them in a later conversation. Or if you find that your needs and your partner's needs arise around the same time, you can learn to gently negotiate and balance both people's needs.

   Since Catherine finds her unmet needs interfere with her ability to meet Fred's needs, the couple can negotiate a plan to balance both their needs. Here is how Catherine can demonstrate sincere consideration to Fred's needs while negotiating her own:

   "I hear what you are sharing, and your feelings are important to me. Though I am overwhelmed, exhausted, and pulled in all directions, I now realize I am trying to manage too much on my own. I want to find a way to spend more time with you. The evenings are hectic, so my suggestion is that you take over bathing the kids and putting them to bed while I clean the kitchen. This will give me some time to shift gears and unwind before you and I come together. I am also open to your suggestions."

   While it is not up to Catherine to figure out the solutions for Fred, she can offer a helpful suggestion. Suggestions are different from solutions, and Fred will also need to be responsible for providing some suggestions that lead to a solution. In this case, Fred (or Catherine) may choose to provide another suggestion like this,

"How about we hire a babysitter once a month so we can go out and spend some time alone together?"

As you can see, a response that includes ownership and curiosity and takes into consideration your partner's needs is more likely to defuse the tension between the two of you. This will also create an opportunity for a productive dialogue that leaves your partner feeling heard and cared for. Moreover, your partner will likely be more receptive to listening to your needs once they feel validated. When both partners feel validated and fulfilled, it can make a world of a difference in the relationship.

IMPORTANT REMINDER: It is vitally important to mention that if you are involved in an abusive relationship, whether it's physical, sexual, financial, verbal or emotional abuse, it will be unlikely for your spouse or partner to change their abusive patterns based only on your changed responses. You may even open yourself up to more abuse or violence. People who are abusive require intensive therapy and anger management tools to stop the abuse and to learn new ways to communicate and behave. ***If you find yourself in an abusive relationship, it is best to seek help from a professional. If you find yourself in immediate danger, I am asking you to please put your safety and that of your child or children at the top of your priority list. If your life is in danger, please call 911, a local crisis line, or a local shelter for victims of domestic violence. I have provided more information on resources in Chapter 6 of this book.***

Contempt

A couple can expect contempt to make its way into the relationship once criticism and defensiveness have become a frequent part of their communication cycle. Contempt is darker than criticism because it comes from a place of lashing out often fueled by feelings of superiority, hopelessness, or a sense of worthlessness in the relationship. Based on

Gottman's research, some examples of contempt present among couples who later divorced were insults, sarcasm, name-calling, hostile humor, mockery, making fun of your partner in front of others, eye rolling, and deep sighing. Typically, couples don't start out by being contemptuous towards each other. Contempt tends to build over time due to unmet bids for connection, one person doing most of the heavy lifting in the relationship, large or small resentments that multiply, forgetfulness, passive-aggressive anger, or a lack of tending to one another.

Let's take a look at examples of how things can escalate from criticism to contempt:

Example 1

Initially: *"Can you please help me around the house? We both live here, so we both need to do our part."*

As time goes on: *"You never help me around the house unless I ask you to do something several times. I'm not your mom, and I shouldn't have to keep asking you and reminding you."*

Eventually: *"There is a pile of dirty clothes sitting in front of you, and you are scrolling through your phone* *look of disgust*. *When are you going to grow up?!"*

Example 2

Initially: *"We need to be careful with our spending if we want to pay off our debt. Let's try to only spend money on what's necessary the next six months."*

As time goes on: *"You keep spending on things that are not necessary. Don't you worry about the debt we have?"*

Eventually: *"You need to get your priorities in check! What's more important, managing our debt or throwing away money on senseless things?* *Sighs and rolls eyes*. *You act like an entitled brat with no sense of responsibility!"*

As shown in the examples above, a criticism can turn into contempt when an issue remains unresolved over a period of time. This often creates a feeling of shame and lack of safety for the recipient of the contempt. When a person feels ashamed and unsafe, they tend to shut down. One thing is for certain: An issue will not suddenly resolve itself through expressing contempt if criticism has already failed to achieve that result. When you are contemptuous towards your partner, not only does it come across as disrespectful, it also conveys a sense of disgust in who they are. In such an atmosphere, you can say good-bye to resolution and hello to more conflict!

Consider a more vulnerable form of communication, such as expressing what is underneath that is fueling the anger and contempt. It will require a dive inwards to understand what is truly upsetting you about a situation—beyond the obvious reason that your partner is not listening to you. Once you are able to identify it, communicate it in a manner that would be more effective. Do your best to be succinct versus going on at length. To help you communicate more effectively so you feel heard and understood by your partner, you can revisit the information on how to express a concern on page 77.

Stonewalling

There is one more common issue Gottman warns couples about: stonewalling. Typically, with enough criticism, contempt, and defensiveness taking place in a relationship, one partner begins to shut down and disengage from the relationship as a way to cope. Like an impenetrable stone wall, this partner sits silently, without making eye contact, nodding, or showing any outward sign of acknowledgement to their critical and/or contemptuous partner. This partner also tends to be the one to withdraw by walking away as conflict rises. While I have seen both genders display stonewalling behavior in my experience working with couples, I have found men more likely to be stonewallers in a relationship.

Imagine this scenario:
Joseph comes home from work. Anna greets him with things she is unhappy about or things he has done wrong. Joseph plops on the couch and turns the TV on, remaining completely silent and appearing to tune out Anna's words. When she probes, he may turn to say, *"okay"* or *"sorry"* but continues to appear expressionless and emotionless, as though he does not care. Other times, he gets up and walks away from her or picks up his phone and tunes her out.

In this scenario, Joseph has stonewalled. Gottman explains stonewalling as a response to feeling flooded (Gottman & Silver, 2000). He refers to flooding as the overwhelming physiological and psychological response felt by a person when they feel attacked, leading to the mind and body eventually learning to shut down, or stonewall, as a way to protect themselves from the flooding sensation. To understand this biologically, the central nervous system becomes activated due to the acute stress a person experiences when they feel attacked, causing a rush of hormones to release in the body, resulting in increased blood pressure, heart rate, and breathing. From an evolutionary standpoint, the body gears up for a fight, flight, or freeze response to perceived danger. Thus, stonewalling can be viewed as a survival response.

Unfortunately, this response makes the other partner feel more desperate to be heard, so they up the ante instead of backing down. This, in turn, causes the stonewalling partner to shut down even more, creating a vicious cycle. If this sounds like your partner, pay attention to how you are approaching them right before they seem to shut down. As outlined in the section on criticism, starting any discussion with a criticism is most likely to result in an unproductive, unresolved, or unresponsive interaction. Instead, consider starting the conversation more gently with your partner, especially around sensitive areas. Find a good time when your partner is less likely to be tired, overwhelmed, or caught off guard and more likely to be open to a discussion. Sometimes, it helps to set a time to talk. When you do find a good time to talk, express your concern—not criticism. Try saying something like this:

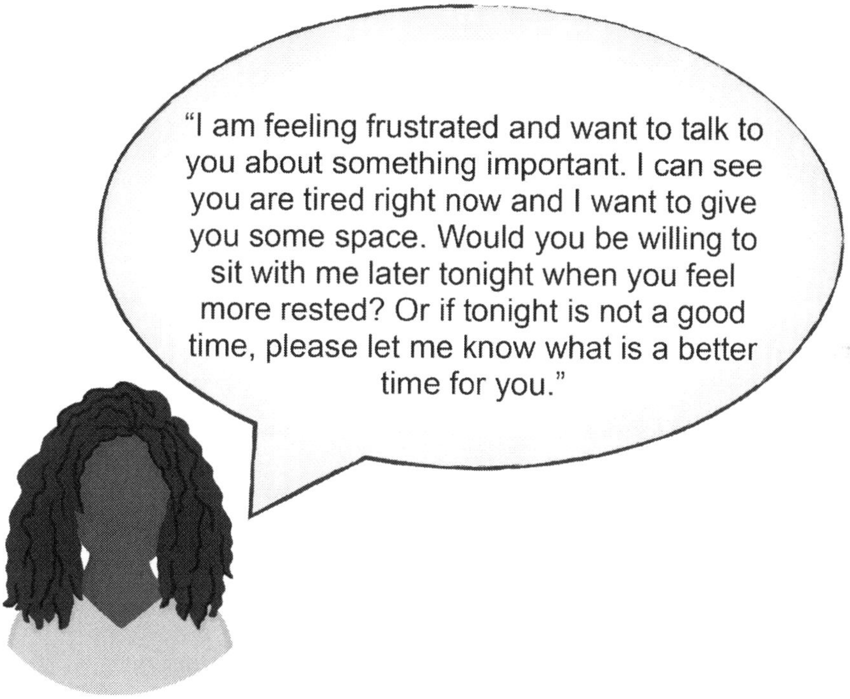
"I am feeling frustrated and want to talk to you about something important. I can see you are tired right now and I want to give you some space. Would you be willing to sit with me later tonight when you feel more rested? Or if tonight is not a good time, please let me know what is a better time for you."

If you are the stonewalling partner, you may be wondering what you're supposed to do instead of shutting down when your partner seems to be angry and attacking you. I recommend developing skills of self-awareness and self-regulation to help you remain present and respond more effectively to your partner. Self-regulation is also an important skill to develop if you are the more critical or contemptuous partner. Continue reading to the next section to learn about emotional regulation, why it's important, and how you can implement it in triggering interactions.

Self-Regulation

Albert Bandura, an influential psychologist in the field of social cognition, originated the self-regulation theory (Bandura, 1991). This theory suggests that humans engage in a dynamic process of personal management to help them decide what to think, feel, say, and do in response to an environmental stimulus, with the goal of becoming the person they want to be. In other words, self-regulation is the process by which you stabilize your nervous system by monitoring and managing your thoughts and emotions. This then helps you choose your response as opposed to reacting out of impulse. Self-regulation is an essential tool for effective communication as you walk into difficult conversations with your partner. It is also a powerful tool for de-escalating heated interactions.

Before I share tips on regulating your emotions to help you manage your reactions towards your partner, I will first provide context from a neurobiological perspective. A simple explanation of neurobiology is learning how the brain and nervous system impact our emotions and behaviors. When you are feeling triggered by your partner, your brain senses danger and sets off alarm bells to alert your body for survival. As a result, the amygdala becomes activated. The amygdala is the most primitive part of your brain and the one responsible for keeping you alive. The amygdala is also part of your limbic system, which is part of the greater nervous system. The amygdala signals your body to release stress hormones to help you fight for survival or run to safety. As such, you are unable to communicate rationally with your partner because your mind and body have entered survival mode.

Once in survival mode, human brains are wired to respond in one of three ways: fight, flight, or freeze. Your survival response can be influenced by what you learned from observing others around you, your attachment style, how you learned to protect yourself from emotional and physical harm, and your natural instincts. It is important to note that your brain is not permanently wired any which way. The more you use it in different ways, it expands and grows—like a muscle! Therefore, you can choose to respond differently in stressful or triggering situations by unlearning old behaviors and learning new ways of responding to your partner. When you repeatedly make a choice on how you would like to respond, it helps to rewire your brain.

Before you can learn to respond differently to a situation, you first have to learn self-regulation skills which will help you monitor your thoughts and manage your emotions. Ultimately, the goal of self-regulation is to stabilize your nervous system. Once your nervous system is feeling calm and centered, your survival instincts will settle down, allowing your left (thinking) and right (feeling) brain to work collaboratively to help you choose your response.

Here are practical steps you can use to self-regulate the next time you find yourself triggered and wanting to fight back or run away:

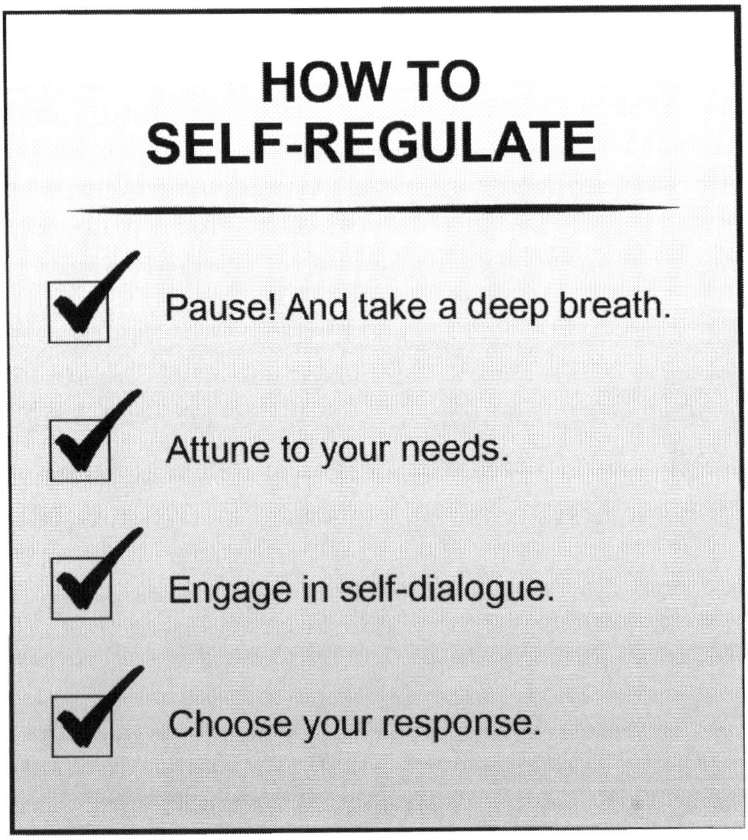
HOW TO
SELF-REGULATE
Pause! And take a deep breath.
Attune to your needs.
Engage in self-dialogue.
Choose your response.

1. **Pause and take a deep breath.** When you start to feel angry, scared, overwhelmed, or reactive in any way—pause. Engage in a mindful breathing exercise. For example, inhale slowly and deeply from your nose for four counts until your belly feels full with air. Next, hold your breath for four counts. Lastly, exhale slowly from your mouth until you count till six. Doing this as many times as you need will stabilize your limbic system where the amygdala is getting ready for a fight-flight-freeze response. Be sure to let your partner know that this is something you will be practicing in difficult conversations.

Try to tune out what your partner is saying for a few moments and focus on yourself. If you need to, and if it feels safe enough to do so, you can let your partner know you need a few moments: *"I am starting to feel* _______ (name emotion) *and I don't want to say something I will regret. Please give me a few seconds."* If you need to step away for a few minutes to regulate, it is okay to do so. Make sure to communicate to your partner why you are stepping away and how much time you need so they don't perceive you as dismissing and walking away. An example of a time-out request can be, *"I want to hear what you are saying, but I am feeling* _______ (name emotion), *and I need a time-out to center myself. I'd like to come back to this in 20 minutes please."*

Deep breathing is one of many mindful grounding techniques you can use to stabilize your nervous system. If you don't find breathing techniques helpful, you can try another mindfulness exercise. For example, look around and identify 10 blue (or any other color) objects in the room. Or engage your five senses by identifying five things you can see, four things you can feel, three things you can hear, two things you can smell, and one thing you can taste. These techniques allow your emotions to settle by shifting your brain's focus towards something else in the present moment.

Another way to help you regulate your emotions is by shifting your attention to another sensation. Some examples are drinking a glass of water, splashing water on your face, and/or feeling something cold with your hands.

2. **Monitor yourself and attune to your needs.** Once your impulse to react fades and you feel calmer, take a moment to decide what you want to achieve from this interaction. Do you want the interaction to escalate where both you and your partner walk away

feeling angry or hurt? Or do you want to come to a resolution where both of you feel heard and understood?

If you want to achieve resolution, continue regulating your emotions and be curious with yourself. Ask yourself what is making you feel upset. Look underneath the anger or the numbness you're experiencing to discover your underlying feelings. Some examples of underlying feelings are fear, overwhelm, rejection, sadness, disappointment, and loneliness. You can revisit Figure 5 on page 51 to understand primary and secondary emotions.

3. **Engage in self-dialogue or self-soothing.** When you are able to identify the underlying feeling(s), engage in a conscious thought process where you name what you are feeling and the possible consequence of reacting to your feeling impulsively. Figure 8 illustrates some examples of what you can say to yourself.

Figure 8

Examples of self-dialogue

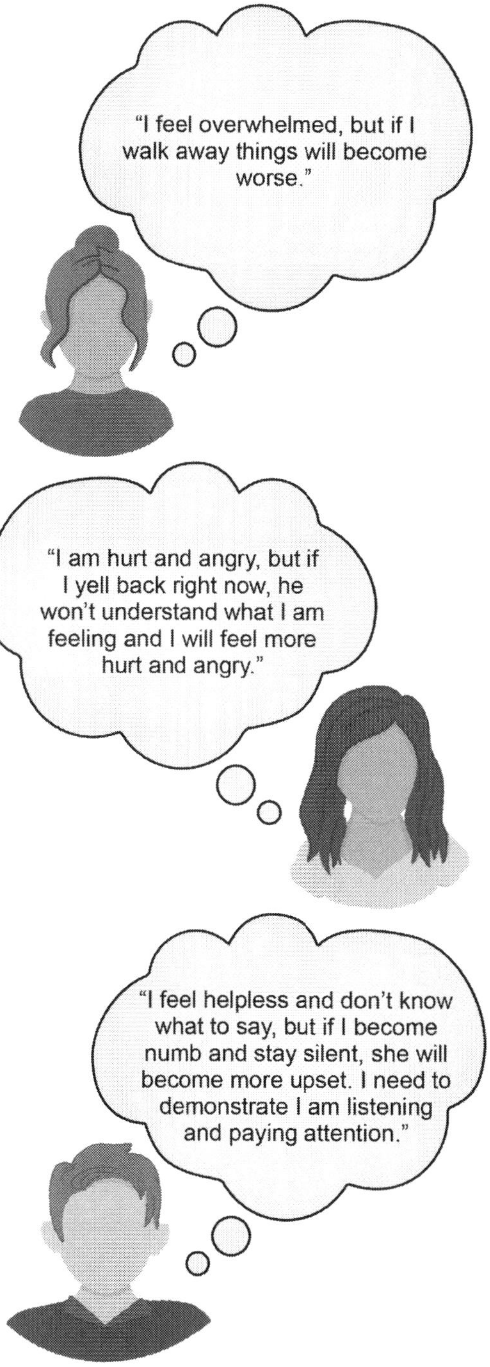
"I feel overwhelmed, but if I walk away things will become worse."
"I am hurt and angry, but if I yell back right now, he won't understand what I am feeling and I will feel more hurt and angry."
"I feel helpless and don't know what to say, but if I become numb and stay silent, she will become more upset. I need to demonstrate I am listening and paying attention."

Some people find it helpful to create phrases, mantras, prayers, or self-affirmations ahead of time so they can remind themselves during triggering situations. When your emotions take over and your brain enters survival mode, your ability to think can be diminished. Therefore, having gentle reminders to refer to can facilitate the process of self-regulation. It can also be useful to note down these reminders somewhere you can easily access them. For example, the reminders can be placed somewhere in the kitchen, on a mirror, on your bedside table, or on your phone. I suggest communicating your intentions to your partner if you plan on stepping away to read these reminders.

If it feels too difficult to access your thoughts during a heated interaction, self-soothing can also be an effective strategy. Self-soothing is any kind of touch which brings you comfort. Some examples include:

- Gently holding your hands or rubbing them together
- Placing your hands on your cheeks
- Touching an object which brings you comfort, such as a ring or necklace
- Feeling something cool or warm around you
- Feeling a different texture, such as your hair, your shirt, or the couch you are sitting on

4. **Choose how you will respond.** Hopefully, you are feeling more regulated after following the first three steps. With increased self-awareness and the ability to think more rationally, explore your options and choose how you would like to respond to your partner. Figure 9 shows a few statements which demonstrate examples of vulnerability and validation in responding to your partner. I talk more about vulnerability and validation later in this chapter.

Figure 9

Examples of vulnerable and validating responses

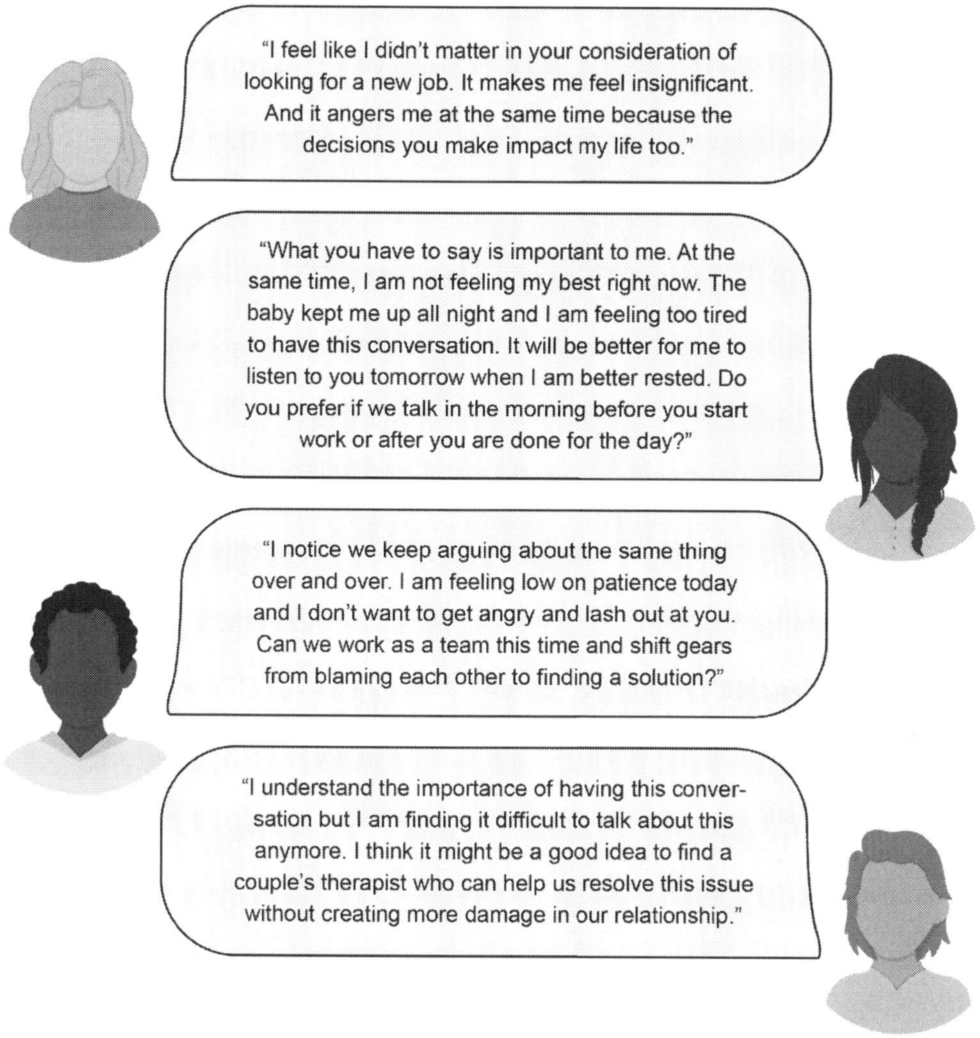
"I feel like I didn't matter in your consideration of looking for a new job. It makes me feel insignificant. And it angers me at the same time because the decisions you make impact my life too."
"What you have to say is important to me. At the same time, I am not feeling my best right now. The baby kept me up all night and I am feeling too tired to have this conversation. It will be better for me to listen to you tomorrow when I am better rested. Do you prefer if we talk in the morning before you start work or after you are done for the day?"
"I notice we keep arguing about the same thing over and over. I am feeling low on patience today and I don't want to get angry and lash out at you. Can we work as a team this time and shift gears from blaming each other to finding a solution?"
"I understand the importance of having this conversation but I am finding it difficult to talk about this anymore. I think it might be a good idea to find a couple's therapist who can help us resolve this issue without creating more damage in our relationship."

To ensure that you maintain a regulated stance, make sure to repeat these steps as needed during a challenging exchange with your partner. You don't have to do all the steps every time you find yourself becoming reactive. Engage in whichever step feels accessible and helpful in the heat of the moment.

Think of self-regulation as a skill to develop. It will not come easily at first. It may feel foreign, uncomfortable, confusing, and even frustrating to some. The important thing to remember is the more you practice this tool, the more naturally it will come to you. Practice regulating your emotions on a daily basis instead of waiting to try it for the first time during conflict with your partner. You can also practice self-regulation when your toddler is making a mess in a room you just cleaned, when your baby is crawling away when you are attempting to change their diaper, when you are facing a stressful day at work, when you are feeling overstimulated, or when you find a pile of dirty dishes in the kitchen sink.

Co-Regulation

Have you ever noticed when someone says "*calm down*" to another person, it can result in the other person becoming more worked up? In fact, you might notice this happens between you and your partner. When either of you tells the other person to calm down, it can make you feel like what you are experiencing is not valid. For this reason, try to avoid statements such as, *"You need to calm down!"* Instead, you can help your partner regulate their emotions by engaging in a process of co-regulation (Butler & Randall, 2013). Co-regulation is the process through which one person, who is feeling more emotionally stable, helps regulate another person who is feeling more overwhelmed with emotion.

Humans have a need for co-regulation as early as infancy (Brumariu, 2015). A baby needs their caregiver to step in and help them regulate their emotions because they are not born with the tools required to cope with distressing experiences. This is true for toddlers and children as well. Children need a loving caregiver to attune to their emotions and help them regulate.

Imagine when a toddler seems to be throwing a tantrum. Tantrums are a sign of the toddler's nervous system being overwhelmed with distressing emotions. When an attuned and responsive caregiver steps in immediately to provide comfort to the child through words, touch, or a soothing presence, it helps the child learn how to regulate their emotions. Thus, co-regulation in childhood develops the skill of self-regulation in adulthood.

Like children, adults sometimes need another person's help to regulate difficult emotions. When you co-regulate as a couple, one partner who feels calmer can help the other partner reach a calmer state. As a matter of fact, even if both you and your partner are feeling dysregulated, you both can help each other move towards a more regulated state. Furthermore, co-regulation not only helps to manage emotions in the moment, it also fosters emotional stability, safety, and a deeper connection between two people in a relationship (Butler & Randall, 2013).

Before you practice co-regulation for the first time, I suggest talking to each other in advance to establish ways to support one another when one or both of you are feeling triggered. In this discussion, it would be wise to explore how you will know if your partner is struggling to self-regulate, how you will communicate the need for co-regulation, how you can suggest a co-regulation technique without escalating the tension, and which techniques you are both willing to try.

IMPORTANT REMINDER: If you are in an abusive relationship, attempting co-regulation may not be safe without the guidance and support of a mental health professional because you may open yourself up to more harm. You are not responsible for causing your partner to act in abusive ways. Abuse of any kind is not okay and never justified. People who are abusive require intensive therapy and anger management tools to stop the abuse and improve their behaviors. ***If you find yourself in an abusive relationship, it is best to seek help from a professional. If you find yourself in immediate danger, I am asking you to please put your safety and that of your child or children at the top of your priority list. If your life is in danger, please call 911, a local crisis line, or a local shelter for victims of domestic***

violence. I have provided more information on resources in Chapter 6 of this book.

During co-regulation, it is paramount to approach your dysregulated partner gently. Remember, you are trying to create a sense of safety so your partner's mind and body can step out of survival mode and return to the present moment. Address your partner using a low, soothing voice, maintain eye contact, keep your body relaxed, and provide a comforting presence.

It is also important to be immediately responsive when you notice your partner finding it difficult to regulate. In other words, help your partner manage their emotions as they are experiencing them. For example, if your partner appears highly anxious and unable to soothe their anxiety, gently step in to help stabilize their nervous system while making sure to keep your own nervous system regulated. If you find yourself becoming agitated while helping your partner, engage in a grounding exercise to maintain balance of your nervous system. You can refer to pages 91 and 92 to review grounding techniques, such as deep breathing.

During co-regulation, you can offer support directly or indirectly in the following three ways:

1. Movement
    - Invite your partner to walk over to a couch to sit with you.
    - Make a suggestion to walk over to a different room before continuing the conversation.
    - Invite your partner to walk with you to the kitchen for a glass of water.
    - Offer to go outside for a walk together.

2. Mindfulness
    - Offer to engage in a deep breathing exercise together.

- Bring your partner's attention to something else, such as the exercise suggested on page 92.
- Share how much you care for your partner to help them attune to the present moment and feel safe.
- Gently remind your partner of a previously agreed-upon mantra, phrase, affirmation, or prayer that helps them feel calm.

3. Touch
    - Sit together quietly and hold hands until you both feel calmer.
    - With consent, engage in a meaningful hug that lasts a few seconds to help decrease stress and increase oxytocin levels, or "love hormones" (Grewen et al., 2005).
    - Bring your partner a previously agreed-upon object which they find soothing, such as a stress ball, a fidget toy, a picture frame of your children, or a sentimental item.
    - Gently remind your partner to feel something cold, such as pressing their hands on the kitchen countertop or holding a glass of water.
    - Offer a shoulder rub or a hand massage.

The suggestions provided above can be adapted to one partner helping the other or both partners helping each other. Some of the ideas might seem unnatural to you; however, they are all simple and effective techniques that can help balance your nervous system. You and your partner can select the ones you feel comfortable trying or research other techniques for co-regulation. As with anything new, it will start to feel more natural the more you do it.

Vulnerability

Why is vulnerability such an uncomfortable thing for most of us? The literal definition of vulnerable is "capable of being physically or emotionally wounded; open to attack or damage" (Merriam-Webster, n.d.). Essentially, when you are vulnerable, you are taking a risk of being hurt. Thus, vulnerability can feel scary, especially if you have been hurt in the past.

That begs the question: Why expose yourself to the risk of being hurt? Because while vulnerability comes with risk, it also comes with an opportunity to build connection. A deeper connection is the ultimate reward of vulnerability in a romantic and co-parenting relationship. When you can learn to be vulnerable, it allows for the possibility of a greater understanding and a stronger connection with your partner.

In my experience, one of the key ingredients couples lack in their communication is the ability to be vulnerable with each other. It seems easier for two people to interact from a place of anger, dismissal, resentment, or avoidance instead of vulnerability. Figure 10 displays a list of reasons why you may find it difficult to be vulnerable with your partner, or any relationship for that matter.

Figure 10

Reasons for lack of vulnerability

1	Growing up, you never saw anyone being vulnerable around you or with you, so you never learned how to be vulnerable.
2	You learned vulnerability is a sign of weakness.
3	You were hurt in the past when you were vulnerable.
4	Due to trauma, it doesn't feel safe to go in your body to experience vulnerable emotions. The vulnerable parts have been shut away.
5	Vulnerability feels scary or uncomfortable to you because it's something you have never tried before.
6	Your feelings have been dismissed, rejected, belittled, or ignored in relationships; therefore, you may have learned to dismiss, reject, and ignore your feelings (common among individuals with an avoidant attachment style).
7	It doesn't feel safe to be vulnerable around certain people because of how they respond to you.

For those of you who are struggling with vulnerability with your significant other, explore why it feels difficult to you. If you notice feelings of confusion, shame, numbness, fear, resentment, or anger, make space for those emotions to teach you where you may have unresolved trauma or pain that could use some attention and healing. Try to address that particular issue whether on your own, with your significant other, or with the help of a therapist. Going to a trained professional is a good idea if you struggle with vulnerability due to trauma, or if you can't seem to overcome the fear or discomfort of vulnerability on your own. Professional help will facilitate insight and self-awareness while teaching you tools to help you heal and grow, leading to increased comfort with being vulnerable in your relationship. Of course, if your relationship is unsafe or domestic violence is present, then safety is always your first consideration.

To be vulnerable in any kind of relationship is an act of courage, whether it is with your parents, children, siblings, friends, significant other, and even yourself. To start somewhere, a good place to practice vulnerability is by understanding *yourself* better. Tune inwards and get to know your vulnerable parts—those parts of you that you feel ambivalent or hostile towards and are afraid to acknowledge, talk about, or accept. Reflect and have honest conversations with yourself. Listen to those parts and attune to their needs because they have something to teach you! Figure 11 shows the type of feelings you may discover as you learn to be vulnerable with yourself and others.

Figure 11

Vulnerable feelings

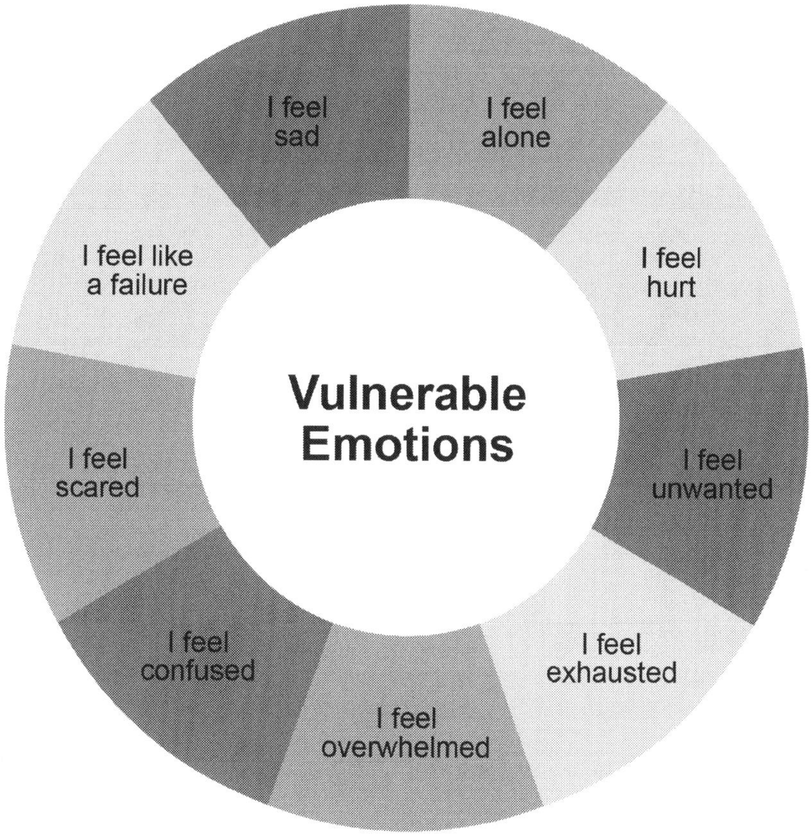
I feel sad
I feel alone
I feel hurt
I feel unwanted
I feel exhausted
I feel overwhelmed
I feel confused
I feel scared
I feel like a failure
Vulnerable Emotions

Once you become more comfortable with being open and honest with yourself, begin to show your vulnerabilities in small ways in a safe relationship. At first, you might feel more comfortable being vulnerable with a friend, a parent, or maybe a co-worker... and that's okay. As you continue to practice, you will know when you are ready to show your vulnerable parts to your significant other as well. You can start with small steps and begin by telling them, *"I can't seem to think straight these days because I haven't slept well for a few nights."* Work your way up to, *"I feel guilty when I yell at the kids and hate myself for it."* Eventually, you might tell your partner, *"I feel like we are growing apart, and that worries me."*

The following example is of a couple where, by the end of the session, the husband, Dave, evolved from communicating harshly to communicating more vulnerably by attuning to his needs:

Michelle and Dave came into their fourth therapy session angry and upset with each other. Having had a baby 14 months prior, they were bravely working through communication challenges with my support. When the session began, Dave explained the couple's argument from the previous evening, sounding resentful and angry. Dave accused Michelle of not responding to his messages for the entire day when he was alone at home caring for their daughter. With shoulders squared off, he blurted out, "She is a selfish person! If she doesn't start acting like she cares about our relationship, then I'm done wasting my time!"

In response to this, a crestfallen and exhausted Michelle explained to me the demanding nature of her job and how disappointed she feels with Dave's lack of understanding and support. She shared how she pulls away from Dave a little bit more each time he picks a fight with her over her inability to respond immediately to his messages when she is at work. When I explored this conflict further with the couple, Dave bravely leaned into his vulnerable parts and shared his insecurities within the relationship. He admitted his fears about Michelle leaving him one day. As we explored the root of these concerns, he connected the dots that he was triggered by her absence from home due to long work hours and frequent work trips. As the conversation continued, Dave revealed he doesn't feel worthy of Michelle, "Some nights I can't sleep thinking she will wake up one day not wanting to spend the rest of her life with me," Dave quietly shared with a deep sigh.

By the end of the session, Dave had shown more vulnerability than ever before in therapy. He spoke directly to Michelle in a more compassionate tone as he said, "I can't see my life without you, Michelle. Sometimes I find myself thinking you will leave me one day, and that scares me. I know it is not right of me to yell at you and say hurtful things because I do understand your work is demanding. What would help me is to know that you will work on prioritizing us more often. Even a small gesture like a text from you in the middle of the day, or to hear you talk about our life together, or for us to plan a weekend away somewhere as a family. I need to feel that you want to be with me as much as I want to be with you... and I'm just not feeling it. I am sorry for the way I have expressed my worries to you. I have used anger and fights to try and feel closer to you, and I am recognizing it's not the right way to handle things."

Michelle quietly listened with tears rolling down her face. After a few silent moments, she said, "I see why you worry about me leaving you. I have been distant from you ever since I started work. After spending a year at home with Ella, it felt good to be away from home—from us. I think working and traveling became my escape. The more we fought about my work, the more I wanted to run towards it. And when I'm home, I just want to be with Ella. If I was in your shoes, I would be worried too. I understand what you're saying. I need to figure out a way to balance work and prioritize my time with you."

For the first time, Dave felt heard. He felt his concerns were taken seriously. In other words, Dave felt validated. With Dave's ability to be vulnerable and Michelle's ability to validate him, the couple's interactions started to change for the better. Both partners began to communicate more vulnerably and respond more compassionately.

Validation is a simple tool which encourages healthy communication between two people, yet it's one I notice couples often struggle with. Let's look at the following section on validation to understand what it is, and what it is not.

Validation

I once had a client who painfully resisted acknowledging his partner's feelings. I finally asked him directly what the resistance was about. He said, "Well I don't agree with what she is saying so I don't know what else to say!" I responded, "You don't have to agree to anything she says to validate her feelings. They are her feelings, and they are real to her, even if you see things differently." To this, he said, "How can I validate without agreeing—that is what validation is, isn't it?"

This client is among many people I work with who have misinformed notions about what validation is. I especially notice a strong resistance among couples to simply sit with and acknowledge their partner's feelings. There is this mistaken belief that to validate means to agree. So, instead of acknowledging how the other feels, I see couples become defensive, dismissive, or begin to offer solutions right out of the gate without understanding what is causing the feeling.

My theory is the defensive, dismissive, and pragmatic responses are due to an inherent misunderstanding that validation is agreement, and to agree would mean one partner has to assume blame for the way the other partner is feeling. Therefore, the best way to avoid blame is to defend yourself, minimize the other's feelings as unsubstantiated or unimportant, or distract from the issue by suggesting a quick fix.

Unfortunately, without validation, the partner who is expressing vulnerably feels unseen, unheard, misunderstood, or not cared about. This can result in the vulnerable partner closing off and putting a wall around to protect them from being hurt again. Or they can hold on to their vulnerable feelings more strongly and express them more loudly, resulting in angry, critical, or contemptuous behaviors. After enough failed attempts hoping to receive their partner's validation, they begin to give up and stop expressing themselves. The negative feelings that develop as a result of this grow silently and deepen over time, eventually leading to a more withdrawn, stonewalling partner.

Some of you might be wondering, "If it isn't agreement, then what is validation?"

Validation is acknowledging your partner's experiences by responding in ways which make them feel seen, heard, understood, and/or cared about. When your partner shares how they feel about something, their feeling is their reality. And a person's reality is often subjective, meaning it's different from yours. For healthy communication to take place, it is crucial to acknowledge your partner's reality as being true for them. And just because it is true for them does not mean it needs to be true for you. You can continue to have your own perspective while acknowledging your partner's perspective.

If you find it difficult to validate your partner's feelings and/or experiences, the best way you can respond is by making a sincere attempt to understand your partner better. Asking questions non-defensively and non-argumentatively is a way of validating because it conveys, *"I hear you, and I see this is important to you. Which makes it important for me to understand and know more about."* Validation can have a powerful impact in bringing two people closer together and deepening their connection.

To help you develop a better sense of how you can validate your partner without necessarily agreeing with their point of view, I have provided examples of validating statements in Figure 12. Notice how most of them convey acknowledgement, not agreement.

Figure 12

Validating statements

- *"That makes sense. If I was in your shoes, I'd feel the same way."*
- *"That sounds awful. I can't believe that was your day!"*
- *"Can you help me understand what is making you resent me right now?"*
- *"Go on, this sounds important. I'm listening."*
- *"I am sorry for how my words came out and how you felt. I didn't mean it that way, but I understand your point of view is different and you're hurting."*
- *"Can you explain what you mean by XYZ? I am having trouble understanding."*
- *"I am sorry. How can I make this right?"*
- *"What can I do right now to help you feel better?"*
- *"I feel sad hearing how you feel. I had no idea you were feeling this way."*
- *"It sounds like XYZ upset you quite a bit. What can I do to meet your needs better so XYZ does not happen again?"*

In summary, validation is not about agreement nor is it about accepting blame. It is about acknowledging your partner's reality as being true for them and important to you. It is also about sitting with your partner's feelings without defending yourself, dismissing them, or offering solutions. Finally, it is about increasing compassion, building connection, and bringing two people closer together.

Pursuer and Withdrawer

You may recall I mentioned in the previous chapter that an anxious and avoidant partnership is the most common type of relationship I observe among couples who come to see me. As it turns out, the two most common communication patterns I witness are also anxious and avoidant. Let's take a look at what the anxious and avoidant communication patterns look like in a heated exchange between two individuals.

Rebecca asks Michael for help with putting their children to bed. Michael says, "*Okay,*" as he continues to respond to a work email on his phone. Rebecca notices he is not helping and feels upset. She asks him for help a second time. Once again, Michael acknowledges her but continues working on his phone. When Rebecca comes back a third time, she is visibly upset and approaches him with a sharp tone: "How can you just sit here and be on your phone while I'm putting both the kids to bed on my own? I've never met anyone as blatantly inconsiderate as you!"

Michael responds with frustration, "What are you talking about? How am I inconsiderate when every day I come home exhausted from work and still play with the kids so you can take a break? Don't you think you are inconsiderate and ungrateful for always complaining about things instead of appreciating what I do for you and our family?!" Michael begins to walk away, infuriating Rebecca. She follows after him, trying to get him to listen to her. She desperately needs him to understand that she is also exhausted from watching the kids all day. She reminds him how she cooks dinner while Michael plays with the kids and how that doesn't count as a "break" for her. She is hoping Michael will turn around and listen to her. Instead, he goes into the basement and bangs the door behind him.

Two hours later when Michael comes back upstairs, Rebecca tries to talk to him again in a calmer tone. Michael tells her he needs to sleep and heads upstairs to their bedroom, quiet and distant from Rebecca. Rebecca feels hurt, alone, and tired. She cries herself to sleep. The next morning, she enters the kitchen and greets Michael, hoping he won't be upset from the night before. Michael responds to her greeting and tries to act normal, but Rebecca senses a coldness about him.

Michael heads to work for the day, and Rebecca does not hear from him until he returns home in the evening. She has spent most of the day replaying their fight from the night before over and over in her head. She feels anxious not knowing what Michael is thinking or feeling. When Michael returns from work, both of them pretend like nothing happened and continue with their regular routine. Rebecca cooks dinner as she watches him play with the kids, anxiously wondering if Michael is still upset with her because he hasn't acknowledged her much.

The interactional cycle between Rebecca and Michael is a common dance between the anxious partner and the avoidant partner in a relationship (Johnson, 2004). As you may have recognized, Rebecca displays an anxious communication style. Dr. Sue Johnson would refer to her as the "pursuer" in the relationship. The pursuer tends to be the one who can escalate conflict by blaming, criticizing and/or attacking their partner. On the other hand, Michael displays an avoidant communication style. He is the "withdrawer" in the relationship, or the one who usually shuts down or walks away from conflict. This partner wants to avoid conflict by any means and can appear closed off.

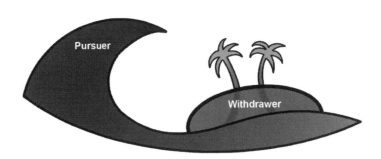
Pursuer
Withdrawer

In this dance between the pursuer and the withdrawer, the more the anxious partner pursues, the more the avoidant partner withdraws, fueling the cycle further (Johnson, 2004). Unfortunately, as was the case between Rebecca and Michael, there is no resolve in this type of a communication cycle. Even though both partners acted normal around each other the following day, Michael continued to be upset, and Rebecca continued to feel hurt and alone. In the absence of resolve and healing, these feelings will be quick to resurface the next time the couple steps into a similar exchange. With each unresolved interaction, feelings will become compounded and leave the couple stuck in this vicious communication cycle.

While Rebecca and Michael's relationship demonstrates the pursuer-withdrawer dynamic, some relationships have two pursuers or two withdrawers. This can happen when the pursuer-withdrawer dynamic evolves over time. The withdrawer can eventually reach their limit and start lashing out at their pursuing partner, or the pursuer can eventually learn their needs will not be met and begin to withdraw like their partner.

No matter what your style of communication is, know that deep down, it is likely you are both hurting in some way. You both probably carry emotional wounds which become triggered in the relationship. What is worse is these wounds deepen each time you engage in a negative communication cycle, like Rebecca and Michael. As a reminder, not all wounds are from the past. Some wounds can be created in your present relationship with each other.

Based on my professional experience, pursuers usually have a pattern of responding to their triggered wound(s) by reaching towards their partner for reassurance, albeit, through blaming, anger, criticisms, and/or anxious energy. This results in pushing their partner further away. On the other hand, withdrawers have a pattern of responding to their triggered wound(s) by distancing or shutting down. Ironically, this results in escalating their partner even more—the very thing they are trying to avoid. If two partners can understand this about themselves and each other, it can develop compassion and facilitate positive change.

In order for change to take place, you first have to become aware of your internal process and understand what is underneath your need to pursue or withdraw. Please review Chapter 2 to help you identify underlying issues which fuel your pursuing or withdrawing behaviors. Without self-awareness, long-lasting, meaningful change is not possible.

Once you attune to your emotions underneath, such as your fears or emotional wounds, and recognize your unmet needs, you can practice communicating more vulnerably. Communicating from a vulnerable place can be an effective way to be heard and understood. As discussed in the earlier section, there is always a risk of being hurt associated with being vulnerable. But there is also a great reward of deepened understanding and stronger connection. Therefore, I will use Rebecca and Michael's story to demonstrate an alternate communication cycle where the two partners are softened and vulnerable with each other:

Rebecca was hot with anger, breathing heavily, and had raging thoughts running through her head as she put her kids to bed alone after asking Michael for help more than once. She felt an urge to release her anger on Michael by giving him an earful about what a selfish and inconsiderate person he was. However, since Rebecca and Michael had started going to therapy together, she was self-aware and mindful of her behaviors. She knew if she went after Michael with anger, he would respond by shifting the blame to her and walking away. She knew this was the moment she needed to regulate herself before approaching Michael.

Once the kids were tucked away, she calmed her nervous system by deep breathing and repeating a mantra with each breath. As she felt the tension leaving her body, she turned inward to understand what made her so angry. As she processed her angry thoughts from a more centered place in mind and body, she was able to identify feeling alone. She felt alone because she believed Michael didn't appreciate the hard work that went into parenting and running a household. She felt he took things for granted and didn't support her enough as a co-parent and as a partner. Rebecca was also able to attune to her feelings of exhaustion and unappreciation. She felt she was self-aware and regulated enough to approach Michael.

Rebecca walked over to Michael, who was still on his phone. Since Michael was also more aware of his patterns and working on improving his communication, he was able to attune to Rebecca's needs and respond adequately. The following is a script which showcases an alternate exchange between the two partners where they use vulnerability and other effective tools for healthy communication learned in therapy:

Rebecca:
"Michael, I am feeling upset about something and hoping to talk to you about it. Will you be free tonight before you go to bed?"

Michael:
"Give me 5 minutes. I need to send out this email for work."

Rebecca puts away the toys in the living room as she waits for Michael, continuing to maintain a regulated nervous system.

Michael:
"Ok, I'm ready. Tell me, what's upsetting you?"

Rebecca:
"Michael, I put the kids to bed on my own tonight. I know this doesn't happen all the time, but it does happen frequently enough where I am starting to feel angry inside. At first, I thought it was because I am exhausted at the end of each day, but I am also realizing it is because I feel alone and unappreciated."

Michael:
"I was tending to an important matter at work. I didn't realize you were feeling exhausted. I thought I usually do pretty well in helping you out when I am home. Can you help me understand your feelings about this?"

Rebecca:
"I know you try to help, but I just don't feel like I get a break. By the time you come home, I am already feeling so tired but instead of resting, I am cooking dinner for everyone. And then you and I both are feeding the kids, giving them showers, and putting them to bed. Even when you are around, I am still thinking and working and caring for everyone. And what upsets me about that is I don't feel like my constant care for everyone in this family is noticed. And that's why I feel alone and unappreciated."

Michael:
"I notice everything you do for us and I do appreciate you. Maybe there is a better way to show it to you. In what ways will you feel appreciated?"

Rebecca:
"I'm not sure… maybe offering to cook or giving the kids a shower without me needing to ask you will help. I think that will make me feel seen and appreciated - like you get how hard my day was and you don't want to take me for granted. It would be nice to sometimes hear you say, 'Hey, go take a break. I'll take care of it!'"

Michael:
"I can do that. I will do a better job of taking more initiative to give you a break and taking on a task."

Rebecca:
"Thank you, that is all I can think of right now. How are you feeling about things? Is there anything I can do better to help you?"

As demonstrated in this interaction, Rebecca practiced self-regulation which helped her communicate more vulnerably with Michael. This made it easier for him to receive what she had to say without becoming defensive, shifting blame, and walking away. Instead, Michael met Rebecca's concerns with curiosity. He chose to validate her by asking her questions non-defensively to understand her feelings better. He also chose to accept responsibility and focus on meeting her needs instead of arguing with her or dismissing her needs. Receiving Michael's validation helped Rebecca remain emotionally regulated and made it possible for her to consider his needs as well.

This form of communication is less likely to trigger wounds as it shifts focus towards vulnerable emotions and subsequent needs. However, if Michael still felt triggered and had the urge to walk away, he could practice self-regulation in order to remain mentally and physically present in the conversation. Michael could say to Rebecca, "Something about this conversation is making it difficult for me to stay present. I am starting to feel overwhelmed. I need to step away for 10 minutes so I can regulate and continue the conversation with you."

In another scenario, if Rebecca had trouble regulating herself and approached the conversation harshly, Michael could say, "I am feeling overwhelmed right now. Can we take a pause and rewind the conversation to start differently? It will really help me if you can let me know what's upsetting you without yelling. Your feelings matter to me, and I want to make sure I am able to stay here with you." Michael could also co-regulate with Rebecca, which would help both of them. As you may recall, co-regulation is the process through which one person helps regulate another person who is feeling emotionally overwhelmed.

After reading this chapter, if you are still experiencing difficulty as a couple in communicating effectively with each other, or you have not been able to identify your emotional wounds and your subsequent needs in the previous chapter, you may find my workshops useful. In these workshops, I provide additional support to couples by helping them gain insight, develop self-awareness, recognize patterns, learn to break patterns, improve communication, and strengthen connection. You can learn more about these workshops by visiting my website: https://www.myottawatherapist.com.

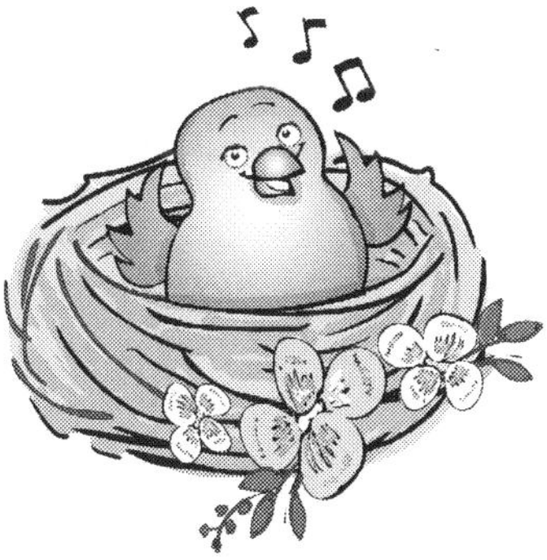

Reflections

What resonated for you in this chapter?

What are the key points you want to remember?

What might be worth discussing with your partner?

What tool or strategy do you want to put into practice?

Chapter 4: *Common Postpartum Struggles Experienced by Couples*

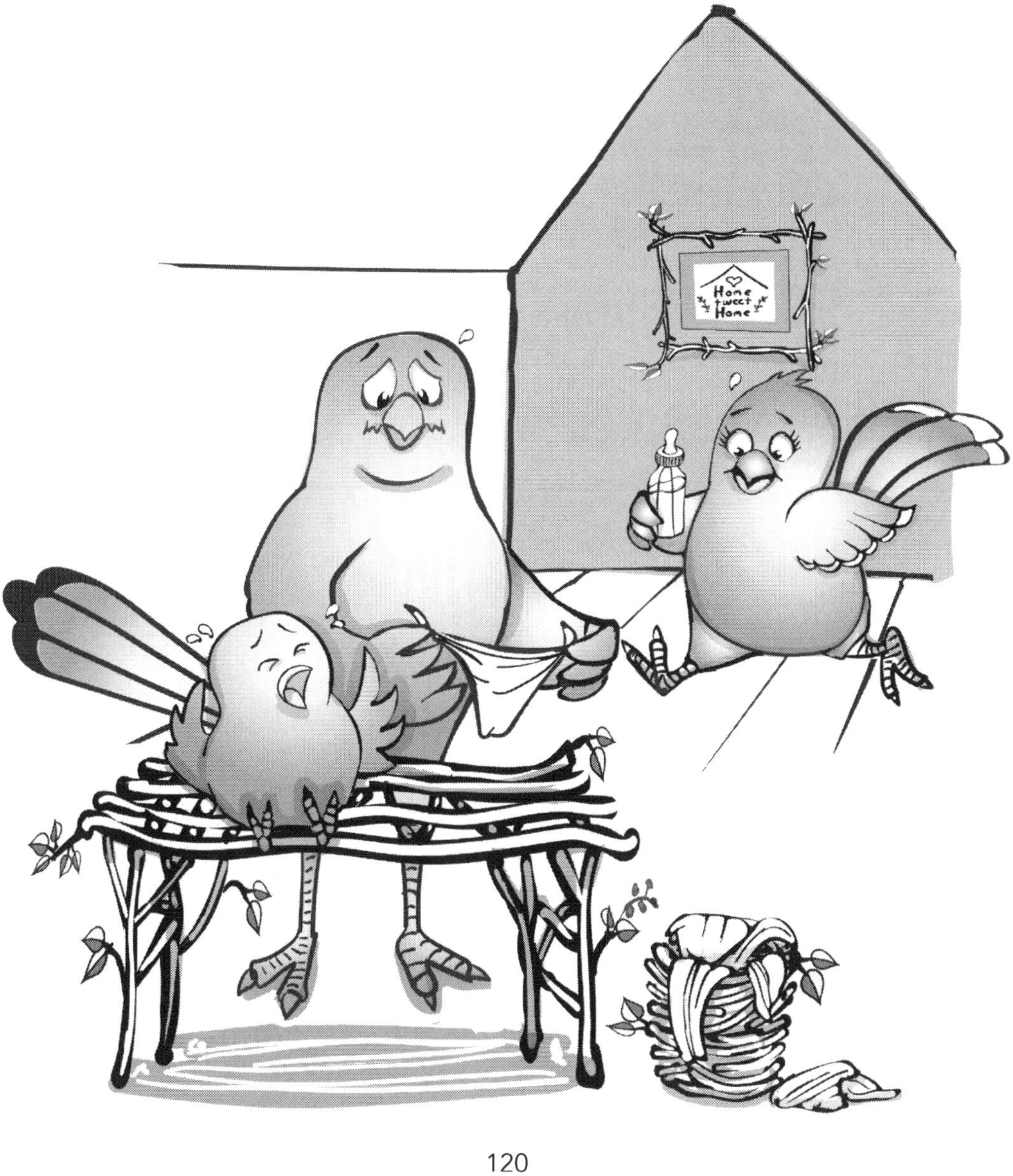
Home
tweet
Home

To Do:

~~Buy baby essentials~~

~~Set up nursery~~

~~20-week ultrasound~~

~~Gender reveal announcement~~

~~Buy dress for baby shower~~

~~Attend prenatal class~~

~~Pack hospital bag~~

Prepare relationship for life after birth

I once conducted an informal survey in 2021 among 63 racially diverse heterosexual couples who were new parents. The majority of these couples were in their thirties, had a college or postgraduate degree, and had an annual household income of $100,000 or more. Among these couples, 16 percent reported experiencing an increase in conflict during pregnancy. This number more than doubled to 43 percent of couples who reported an increase in conflict during the first three months postpartum.

Why is that?

Transitioning to parenthood is a difficult chapter for most new parents—and a topic that is talked less about. Very few couples are prepared for the dramatic shift that takes place in their lives with the arrival of their firstborn. Long gone are the lazy Sundays, date nights, and spontaneous plans with friends. Life in those first few months after baby becomes about survival. Your focus is on trying to get through each day after every sleepless night while also learning to care for a little one who is completely dependent on you for their own survival.

Amidst all of this, a couple transitions from being partners in a relationship to parents of a newborn baby overnight. Couples step into the new role of parenthood without having the time to process the drastic changes: from lack of sleep, energy, intimacy, and time alone, to an overload of responsibilities, exhaustion, and family time—grandparents included! With all these changes that impact a couple's relationship, it is no surprise that 67 percent of couples report a decline in their marital satisfaction for as much as three years after having their first child (Shapiro, Gottman, & Carrère, 2000). This research also supports the findings of my own survey as mentioned above.

Specific to my survey, I asked questions related to experiences during pregnancy and the first three months postpartum. The three most common emotions both mothers and fathers described during pregnancy were happiness, nervousness, and excitement. On the other hand, the three most common emotions both mothers and fathers described during the first three months after birth were feelings of overwhelm and exhaustion along with happiness and love. As displayed in Figure 13, the couples also shared common thoughts associated with their emotions during pregnancy and postpartum.

Figure 13

Common thought patterns among new parents

Common Thought Patterns

	Pregnancy	Postpartum
New Mothers	• Concerns about whether their baby will make it to full term • Fear around labor and delivery • Wondering what type of parent they will be	• Questioning their capabilities as a mother • Concerns about challenges related to breastfeeding
New Fathers	• Wondering about the future and whether they can provide adequately for their family • Concerns about their partner's health and how to best support them	• Uncertainty around how to help and support their partner
Both Parents	• Concerns about their baby's health • Excitement to meet their baby and about the future • Wondering if they are ready to be parents	• How much love and gratitude they feel • How tired and overwhelmed they are

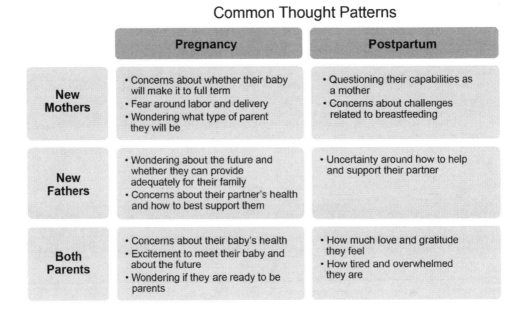

Note: Results from survey conducted by Zara Arshad (2021)

These findings shed light on the internal experiences of each partner and give context to reasons why there might be increased conflict or dissatisfaction in a relationship after the birth of a child (or children). It also explains why young couples come to see me after recently having had their first baby. Not surprisingly, most of these couples describe increased conflict and an inability to communicate effectively as their reason for seeking professional help. While there are unique experiences in every relationship, I have come to recognize 10 common areas of conflict between partners who are new parents. I will expand on each of these areas in this chapter.

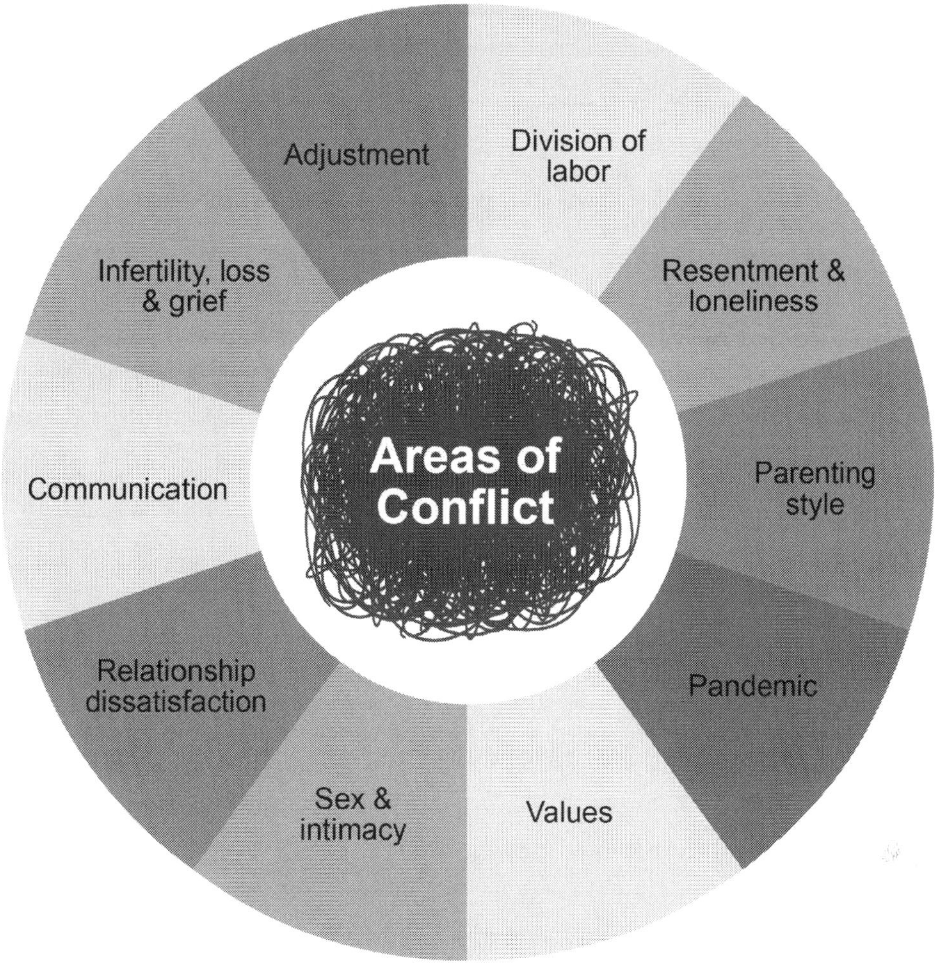
Adjustment
Division of labor
Resentment & loneliness
Parenting style
Pandemic
Values
Sex & intimacy
Relationship dissatisfaction
Communication
Infertility, loss & grief
Areas of Conflict

Adjustment

Life changes drastically with the birth of a child. As a new parent, you are likely discovering it can be overwhelming the first few weeks or months trying to adjust to what has become your new normal. What does the new normal entail?

Notably, the biggest difference is where you once lived life according to your own terms, you now live on the terms of the little bundle snuggled up in your arms (or screaming in the crib!). The needs of your newborn baby largely include nourishment, comfort, safety, and sleep. Therefore, the new normal becomes a never-ending cycle of sleepless nights, feeding, burping, soothing your baby, rocking them to sleep, washing their bottles, doing their laundry, and a whole lot of diaper changes!

In addition to the typical demands of caring for a newborn, some parents experience unique stressors related to managing their baby's physical health from the moment their child is born. These parents have babies who were premature at birth, have acid reflux, are colicky, are not gaining weight, are unable to latch on to breast or bottle, have an abnormality since birth, or have any other physical and health-related complications. Some of these parents have to spend several weeks, even months, at the hospital as their baby is looked after in the neonatal intensive care unit (NICU). Others have to schedule numerous appointments to meet with doctors and specialists.

Finally, on top of everything else, mothers endure the pain and discomfort of physical recovery after birth while learning to care for their baby at the same time. Some of these mothers have also experienced trauma during or after birth which impacts their mental health. Others experience postpartum mood disturbances. Between the physical and emotional recovery of the birthing parent, the sudden load of new responsibilities, and the shift in the couple's relationship from partners to parents, a roller coaster of emotions can also become the new normal:

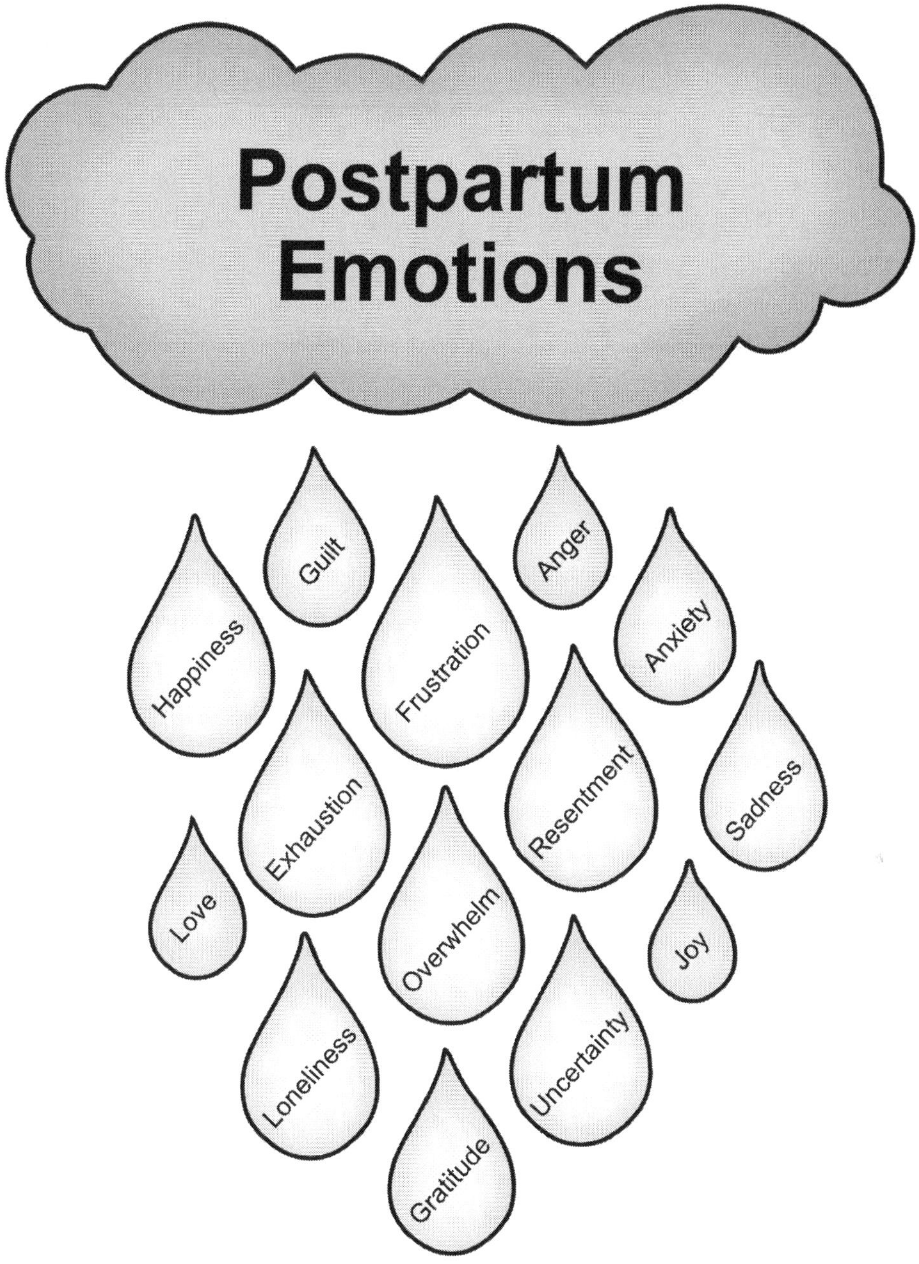
Postpartum
Emotions
Guilt
Anger
Happiness
Frustration
Anxiety
Exhaustion
Resentment
Sadness
Love
Overwhelm
Joy
Loneliness
Uncertainty
Gratitude

In the first few weeks after birth, conversations between the couple largely revolve around figuring out how to take care of their baby, what needs to be done around the house, and how responsibilities will be divided or shared. Though this is not the case with every couple or parent, many times it is the mother who takes time off from work to stay home with their baby. For the stay-at-home mother, the new reality also includes less time and fewer opportunities to complete important tasks, take care of their health, leave the house any time they want, engage in social activities with friends or family, have time alone, enjoy hobbies, or meet the demands of anything else going on in their life aside from parenthood. These factors could explain why new mothers experience problems more intensely than their partners and why they display decreased conflict management skills (Doss et al., 2009).

Another factor that can influence adjustment for new parents is the length of maternal and paternal leave. Some countries, like Canada, allow the opportunity for long paid leaves to both mothers and fathers. However, other countries, such as the United States, don't provide the same benefits or opportunities to new parents. In such countries, working mothers hardly have the opportunity to adjust to life with their newborn before they have to return to work. Mothers who don't have the option to quit their job, or the ones who don't want to, can experience mixed emotions such as stress, guilt, relief, anxiety, happiness, grief, confusion, and sadness. These emotions are about their return to work, leaving their newborn in someone else's care, and the difficulties of trying to create work-life balance so they can have more time and energy for their baby.

Breastfeeding mothers experience additional challenges as they try to maintain a pump schedule at work in order to keep up their milk supply. These mothers can face logistical issues at their workplace on a daily basis and the frustrations that come with trying to navigate these issues. The experience can be exacerbated if their place of employment is not respectful, supportive, or accommodating of breastfeeding mothers.

Mothers who have the option to quit work or the ones who have the opportunity to take a long maternity leave also experience a mix of emotions around their decision to stay home with their baby. While these mothers can feel grateful to be close to their baby, some of them also experience negative emotions due to loss of connection with people, independence, their ability to leave home, opportunities, and growth in their career. The decision to stay home can also have financial repercussions which can impact a couple's relationship, especially if a partner was not in agreement with the mother's decision.

Stay-at-home mothers who don't have support, understanding, or appreciation from their partner or from other adults in their life find it more difficult to adjust in their new reality. In my therapy sessions, mothers describe feelings of exhaustion, anxiety, isolation, resentment, loneliness, and/or burnout. Among the Canadian mothers I helped in my practice during 2020-2022, many have attributed exacerbated negative feelings and conflict in their relationship to the COVID-19 pandemic. These mothers are the ones who gave birth to a child before the start or during the pandemic. Research also supports significant increases in anxiety and depression in maternal mental health since the start of the pandemic (Kotlar et al., 2021).

By now, some of you might be wondering,

"*Where is the hope in all of this?!*"

"How do we manage having a good relationship after children?"

"Is it possible to get back to the relationship we once shared?"

While couples do experience challenges in their relationship after having children, things start to settle for most parents over time. Think of it as a journey you have to navigate together. In this journey, you begin to understand your children's needs better, develop manageable routines, learn to communicate more effectively, sort out roles and responsibilities, seek support, learn new tools to manage your mental health, figure out parenthood, learn to accept the new normal, and find ways to maintain or redevelop the connection you share as a couple. Some of this occurs naturally where things begin to fall into place over time as a couple makes adjustments based on trial and error. Other areas require conscious awareness, flexibility, compromise, negotiation, and a sincere effort towards positive change.

However, with physical, mental, and emotional energy depleted after having a baby, it can be hard to reflect on what the issues are and what changes need to be made. Even if a couple makes it this far in becoming aware, they might struggle to figure out how to create change in the relationship. If you find yourself unable to create necessary changes on your own, consider reaching out to a couple's therapist who specializes in perinatal mental health. You don't have to suffer alone, nor do you have to figure it all out on your own. It is appropriate to seek professional help, and it is wise to do so in a timely manner. I have included professional resources in Chapter 6 of this book as support.

When postpartum couples come to me for relationship help, I notice how some of them express frustrations or dissatisfaction when their partner doesn't meet their expectations. A couple does not necessarily come into the first session articulating their issues as one of unmet expectations. Usually, this is a pattern I come to discern as they describe their arguments or disappointments.

These expectations could be spoken or unspoken. They are typically centered around childcare, household chores, and providing emotional or physical support to one another, especially the parent primarily responsible for the childcare. If you are recognizing tension in your relationship due to unmet expectations, reflect on whether you have clearly shared what your expectations are and how you have communicated them. Upon reflection, you might realize you have not clearly shared your expectations with your partner. Or you have communicated them through criticisms or harsh remarks. As you may recall, criticisms and harshness never bode well for a conversation—or a relationship. It is also possible that one or both of you may be struggling to meet the other's expectations. Rather than clearly communicating this, you or your partner may be reacting with hostile, defensive, or distanced behaviors.

As you adjust to your new normal, it might become necessary for you and your partner to manage your expectations of each other. Here are a few ways you and your partner can support each other better and reduce the likelihood of conflict resulting from unmet expectations:

1) If you have not had your baby yet, before or during pregnancy is a great time to open up dialogue around what each of you is imagining life will be like after your baby is born. Talk to each other about your life right now, what your roles and responsibilities look like, and where both of you will need to make adjustments once your baby arrives. This is also a great time to share any expectations you have of each other as future co-parents to your baby. As you engage in this conversation, it would be wise to remember that reality might be different than what you're expecting after your baby is born. Therefore, flexibility and openness to changes will be important for healthy adjustment.

   The following are questions you can ask each other to prepare your relationship for life after birth:

- What expectations do you have of me currently as your wife/husband/partner?
- How do you think your expectations will change, or remain the same, after our baby arrives?

- What expectations do you think you will have of me as a mother/father to our child?
- After our baby arrives, what roles and responsibilities do you expect me to:
  - ✦ Maintain
  - ✦ Take on
  - ✦ Let go of
- What changes do you anticipate in our relationship after we become parents?
- What is your hope for us as a couple as we transition to parenthood?
- How are you imagining our life in the first few weeks postpartum?
- What do you think our days will look like?
- What do you think our nights will look like?
- What kind of support are you expecting me to give you?
- What happens if reality is different than our expectations?
- How can we manage the tension between expectation and reality?

Remember to utilize communication tools you learned in Chapter 3 as you ask each other these questions, such as vulnerability, validation, asking questions non-defensively, listening to understand (instead of reacting or debating), regulating your emotions, and working as a team. If you are interested in reading more on the topic of expectations, you can take a look at Chapter 5 where I dive deeply into explaining the impact of unmanaged expectations.

2) If you have already had your baby, find a good time when both of you are in the right mental space before bringing up any relationship or parenting concerns. In the first few weeks postpartum, each of you might be feeling overwhelmed and exhausted. For this reason, it will be crucial to have important conversations when both of you have the mental capacity to listen and engage responsively. Consider setting up a time beforehand instead of springing the conversation on each other.

   Once you both find a good time to talk, engage in an open dialogue approached with curiosity to understand each other's experiences. Address each other as members of the same team who want to work together and help each other succeed. Talk about the roles and responsibilities both of you share, who needs help where, how can each partner support the other better, and what are a few things both of you are willing to work on. Maintaining a healthy relationship while transitioning to parenthood requires sincere effort, patience with yourself and your partner, good communication, flexibility, and a willingness to hold yourself accountable and change.

3) Do weekly check-ins with each other in the first few months postpartum. During the check-ins, discuss what is working and what is not working using the communication skills you have learned in this book. Remember, harsh startups or criticisms won't make it easy for your partner to be open to what you have to say. It will put them on the defensive where they will feel the need to either attack back or walk away from you. Continue working as a team and be willing to modify roles and responsibilities to improve as co-parents and to help support each other better.

Gentle reminder that this is a practice and not an exercise in perfection. With lack of sleep, overwhelm, and exhaustion being the new normal in life after birth, new parents can find it difficult to communicate kindly and respectfully with each other. Frustrations can rise despite your best efforts of implementing good communication strategies. This is completely normal and expected even in the healthiest of relationships. If you step into an angry exchange of words with your partner, take some time to reflect and become aware of what is underneath your anger and what it is you need. Once you recognize your underlying emotion and the subsequent need, turn to your partner with the intention of making amends by approaching them from a softer, more vulnerable stance. If you are having trouble understanding or applying any of these concepts, it may help you to review the sections on identifying emotional needs as well as ruptures and repairs in Chapter 2.

To showcase how a couple can use good communication skills to figure out ways to adjust to their new normal together, I have presented the following dialogue between Yasmin and Firouz, a married couple who gave birth to their son three months ago:

THURSDAY

YASMIN:
I'm feeling exhausted lately.
Can we talk today?

FIROUZ:
I'm really tired today. How about we talk on Saturday when I have more energy?

YASMIN:
Saturday works for me. We can talk when Ali is taking his nap.

FIROUZ:
Okay, I'll put a reminder in my phone so I don't forget.

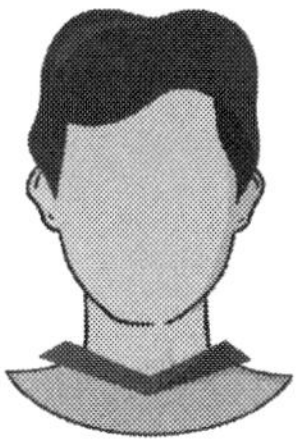

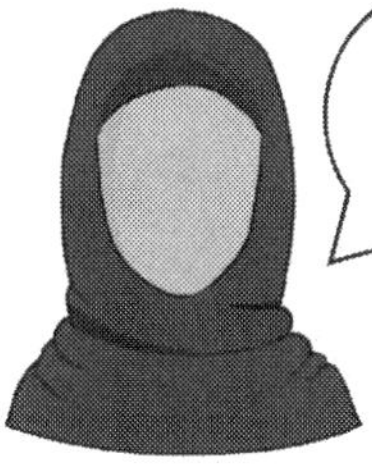

YASMIN:
Thank you!

SATURDAY

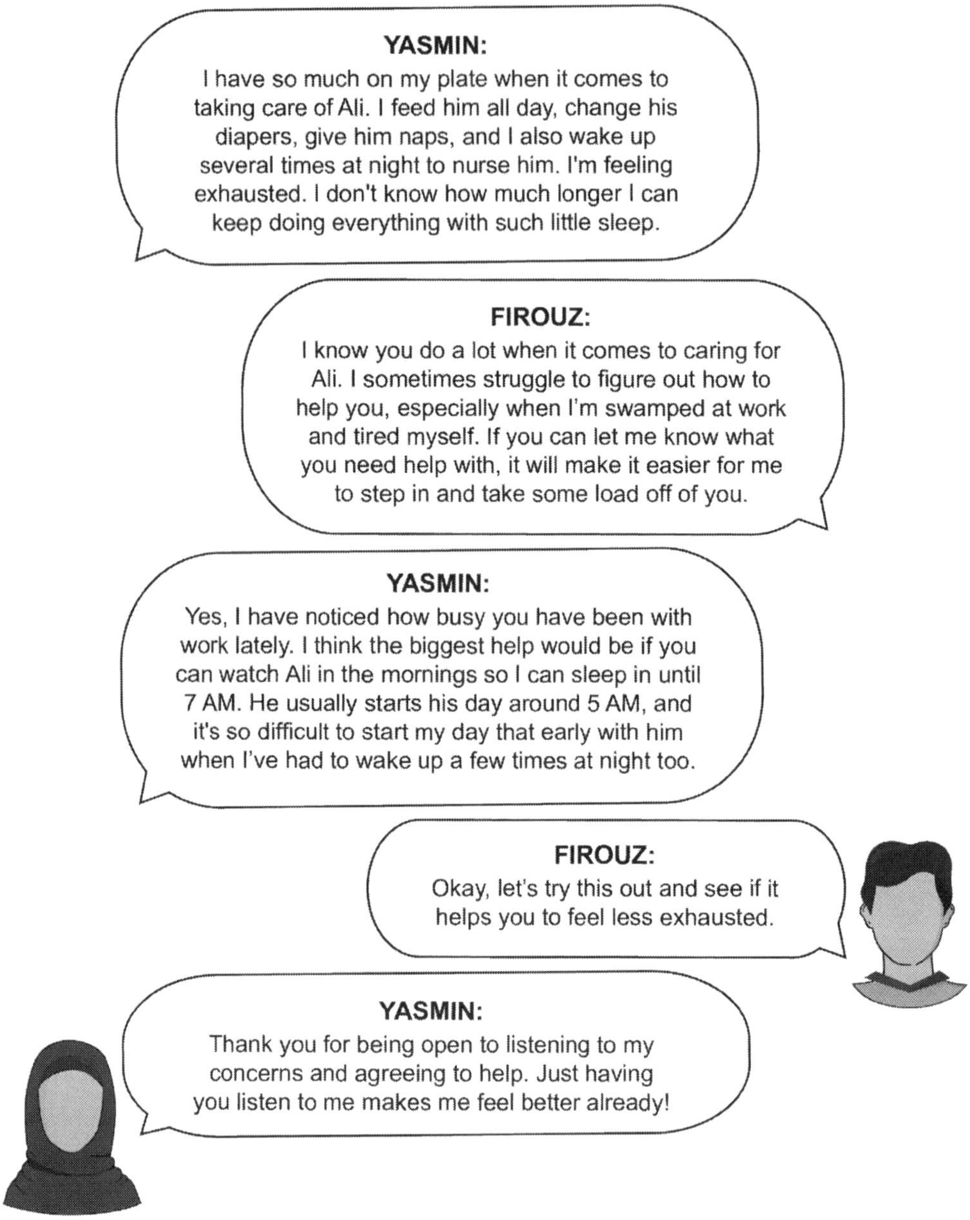
YASMIN:
I have so much on my plate when it comes to taking care of Ali. I feed him all day, change his diapers, give him naps, and I also wake up several times at night to nurse him. I'm feeling exhausted. I don't know how much longer I can keep doing everything with such little sleep.
FIROUZ:
I know you do a lot when it comes to caring for Ali. I sometimes struggle to figure out how to help you, especially when I'm swamped at work and tired myself. If you can let me know what you need help with, it will make it easier for me to step in and take some load off of you.
YASMIN:
Yes, I have noticed how busy you have been with work lately. I think the biggest help would be if you can watch Ali in the mornings so I can sleep in until 7 AM. He usually starts his day around 5 AM, and it's so difficult to start my day that early with him when I've had to wake up a few times at night too.
FIROUZ:
Okay, let's try this out and see if it helps you to feel less exhausted.
YASMIN:
Thank you for being open to listening to my concerns and agreeing to help. Just having you listen to me makes me feel better already!

In this exchange, Yasmin is aware of how she is feeling and what it is she needs. From experience, she knows Firouz will become angry and defensive if she begins a conversation with a harsh start-up by blaming him or criticizing him for something. Instead, she approaches her husband using "I" statements. She maintains focus on what *she* is struggling with and what *she* needs help with instead of pointing fingers with "you" statements, such as "You don't help me." As a result, Firouz is able to stay present, listen to what she is saying, and respond to her needs non-defensively. Both of them speak vulnerably and respectfully with each other, acknowledging their own challenges and limitations while also validating the other's experiences.

As I close on the topic of adjusting to your new normal, I am hoping your biggest take away is to recognize the importance of maintaining or developing a strong partnership when a baby is born. It is a team effort and requires both partners to put their best foot forward to support each other. While having your first baby brings excitement and joy, it is also a steep learning curve—for both mothers and fathers. Each partner faces their own challenges, and each requires help in different ways. Practice working together as a team to figure out what will create a strong partnership as you transition to becoming a family with children.

Division of Labor

A fairly common argument I observe happening in sessions is the age-old question: Who does more?

Amber and Tony came into every session arguing about who does more work than the other. If I did not stop them, they would easily spend each therapy hour going back and forth on who does all the work with the kids, who does all the work in the house, whose job is more difficult, who stays up more at night, who is more tired, and so on.

They found themselves so stuck on the topic of division of labor that it took several sessions to be able to get to a place where they were able to appreciate each other and recognize the role each partner plays to take care of their family. Notably, it was usually Amber who would throw the first jab at how she does everything between taking care of their children, cooking, and working, among many other tasks she would list out. In response, Tony would become frustrated and respond defensively, explaining how he bathes the kids and puts them to bed, he watches the kids after school so she can cook dinner, and he does all the yard work.

Every now and again, Tony would also highlight how he is the one who is "always" trying to be upbeat and happy for the family while she is "always" angry and yelling. Amber would typically respond by icily reminding Tony she would not be angry if he did more to help her. By this point, Tony would be flustered, red in the face, and throw his hands up in the air as though there was nothing he can say or do that would ever make his wife appreciate him.

In Amber and Tony's case, Amber perceives herself as the primary parent while also being a working professional. What do I mean by primary parent? This is the parent that feels responsible for nearly all aspects of the children's well-being. This is also the parent that takes on the invisible labor of parenthood. The invisible labor is all the intangible things the parent does and the load they carry in their mind: the mental notes, trackers, lists, questions, information, appointments, and decisions. These are all the things the other parent—or anyone for that matter—cannot see, hear, or feel but that are as important as the more tangible, physical load of parenthood: giving a bath, rocking baby to sleep, feeding milk, cooking dinner, changing diapers, and so forth.

Invisible Labor of the Primary Parent in the First Year

- Anticipating and attuning to baby's needs
- Implementing a schedule for the baby
- Creating & implementing a nap routine
- Tracking baby's sleep & hunger cues
- Planning separate meals for the baby & the family
- Researching sleep training methods
- Remembering to order more diapers before they run out
- Ensuring baby's clothes & belongings are washed
- Ensuring baby has adequate rest & play time
- Attuning to baby's preferences in terms of comfort, sleep, play, and food
- Researching doctors & specialists
- Managing appointments
- Taking baby to their appointments
- Noting down questions for the pediatrician
- Tracking baby's height & weight
- Managing baby's medications & health needs
- Knowing baby's clothing size
- Remembering to purchase seasonal gear for baby
- Tracking milestones
- Planning baby's first birthday
- Sharing updates with the family

Amber found herself to be aware and attuned to everything when it came to the care of her two children. Even when she was away from home, she felt responsible for keeping track of several things throughout each day that were related to childcare. She found herself exhausted and on edge around Tony and the children. Tony did not understand why she was angry because he perceived himself contributing equally to the care of their children. Based on the things Amber would describe, she performed the invisible labor of motherhood. For example, even though Tony cooked dinner on the days Amber worked late, Amber would have to remember to text him at some point during her workday to let him know what to cook for dinner. This is because she was the one who had planned meals for the week and had done the groceries ahead of time to make sure the children had fresh and nutritious meals.

Similar to Amber and Tony's situation, I have observed this dynamic among other couples where one partner plays the role of the primary parent. In my experience living and working in a Western society, it has often been the mothers who play this role, even in the case of the ones who are working. I have noticed women tend to assume the role of primary parent whether it is naturally, reluctantly, happily, begrudgingly, or with mixed emotions. Of course, this is not true of all couples. This is simply a pattern I have noticed among couples who come in to see me in my therapy practice.

So how does the issue of division of labor show up in my work with parents of small children? Here is an example of what Amber and Tony shared with me during a session: Amber asked Tony to put away the dishes; she expected this task to be done soon. A few minutes later when she saw Tony laying on the couch with dirty dishes still sitting in the sink, she approached him with anger. Tony immediately returned the anger by becoming defensive. When the argument escalated, Tony got up from the couch and left the room. Amber put away the dishes herself as she simmered with angry thoughts towards her husband.

When a couple shares a scenario like this, I might ask them to give me a few more examples. With each example they share, I go below the surface with them and help them identify what is fueling the conflict in each scenario. This helps my clients recognize that while each argument appears to be about different topics, there is a similar underlying pattern.

In Amber and Tony's example, Amber recognized that her anxiety is usually present before she even asks Tony to do something. This is because a part of her always predicts that whatever she is asking of him either won't be done or it will not be done well. She believes this to be true because she thinks Tony takes her for granted and expects her to do everything. In the case of the dirty dishes, she was already feeling anxious with these negative thoughts before she asked for his help. Hence, seeing Tony lying down with the dishes still in the sink was enough to tip her over; it affirmed her anxious thoughts as being valid.

As Tony reflected on his own underlying process, he discovered a familiar feeling which came with his wife's frequent disappointment in him. He recognized his pattern of avoidance and/or disinterest in helping her because he felt he could never live up to her standards. Whether or not he did what Amber asked of him, he would feel that familiar feeling of disappointment inside when she would approach him critically or harshly. He was tired of feeling this way; therefore, he now resorted to angrily defending himself and walking away. Other times, he became passive aggressive by ignoring her or dragging his feet if she asked for help.

Unfortunately, every time Tony walked away or became passive aggressive, Amber felt dismissed or belittled, and it deepened the feelings of resentment inside of her. Not only did she feel exhausted between childcare, work, house chores, and carrying the invisible load, she also felt alone and taken for granted. She believed Tony did not appreciate the physical and mental load she carried in taking care of their family. Because of these built-up feelings, she got in the habit of engaging in negative thought patterns frequently, which only aggravated her anxiety.

Through identifying these patterns, it became clear that Amber carried feelings of anxiety, exhaustion, loneliness, and resentment underneath her anger. Since Amber had not yet learned the tools to communicate these feelings, Tony only witnessed her anger and criticisms during conflict. As a result, he started to believe he was a disappointment to her. On the other hand, Amber was not aware of how hurt Tony felt inside because she only witnessed him being defensive and walking away from her.

Fortunately, as the couple gained new insights by discovering underlying patterns in therapy, they were able to understand each other better. They were also able to recognize that they were not in conflict about the dirty dishes (or whatever the topic in question may be), rather, they were in conflict about the pain they both carried inside. This helped them develop enough compassion towards each other to warrant a shift in their conversations. They made conscious efforts to break old patterns of hurting each other and develop new ones to help one another feel loved and appreciated. Thus, instead of arguing about who did more, they engaged in meaningful conversations around how they could appreciate and support one another better as partners, co-parents, and teammates.

Like Amber and Tony, couples experiencing conflict over division of labor are typically stuck in unhealthy cycles of anger, blame, and defensiveness. When this is compounded with sleep deprivation, fatigue, the toll of caring for your baby, physical recovery, and postpartum mood disturbance, the impact can be significant on a couple's mental health and on the quality of their relationship.

If there is conflict in your relationship regarding division of labor, it is time to take a step back and become introspective about what is fueling the tension. While it may appear to be about childcare duties and house-related chores, the tension may have more to do with prolonged feelings of loneliness, resentment, and unappreciation. To help you discover underlying patterns, become self-aware, and develop new perspectives, reflect on the following questions:

- What feelings come up when I think my partner is not doing enough to help?
- What feelings come up when my partner criticizes me for something I did or didn't do?
- What do I tell myself when my partner does not help me, or does not help me adequately?
- How do I feel about the way our roles and responsibilities are currently divided?
- Why do I feel this way? What do I think needs to change?
- What are some common thoughts and feelings I have during conflict around roles and responsibilities?
- Is my partner truly aware of how I feel inside?
- How can my partner better support me? Have I communicated this to my partner, and in what manner?
- Am I doing enough to appreciate my partner and support them better?
- Have I put myself in my partner's shoes? Do I truly understand them?

While we are on the topic of division of labor, it is important to point out the different expectations among couples of different cultural backgrounds. Strict gender role ascriptions are prevalent in many patriarchal societies globally and are practiced widely, including in North America. Regardless of which culture you identify with, it is important to evaluate what is working and what is not working between you and your partner. As a couple, you may decide you would like to split all roles and responsibilities relatively 50-50 including work, childcare, chores, errands, and other tasks. Or the two of you may decide to split things differently based on what seems acceptable and reasonable to you. What is acceptable and reasonable to you may be influenced by your cultural values, beliefs, and practices. If your current division of labor isn't causing feelings of distress, dissatisfaction, or disconnection in your relationship, then there may not be any need for changes.

On the contrary, if you find that the current division of labor in your partnership is impacting your mental health and your relationship, it might be time to open up the discussion with your partner. In the case where one of you expects more traditional gender role practices and the other expects more egalitarian practices, ask each other questions to understand one another better before jumping to defending your position. Find out why it is important for each of you to implement or maintain the different types of gender role practices. As a result of mutually respectful, curious, and open conversations where both of you feel heard and understood, you may find it easier to compromise and negotiate your roles and responsibilities.

If it helps, you can also think of your relationship as a business partnership for a few months. I know it doesn't sound very romantic but, truth be told, those few months after having your baby are mostly about survival. Therefore, it may help to think of yourselves as two partners learning how to run a new business successfully. Consider having weekly meetings where you come together as a team to re-evaluate your roles and responsibilities in order to improve running your business. Start each meeting with appreciating one another for all that you do, identify what is working and what is not working, discuss your strengths and weaknesses, and agree upon any desired changes. This is not to suggest that romance is not important; rather, it is a creative suggestion to consider in order to support each other better during the early stage of new parenthood.

For those couples who become reactive and tend to escalate, I recommend establishing ground rules for these meetings ahead of time so you both approach each meeting with the same mindset. Make sure to establish a rule for when things become heated and there is a need to pause and regulate emotions before continuing. Here is a suggestion of three steps both of you can agree to follow if emotions begin to rise:

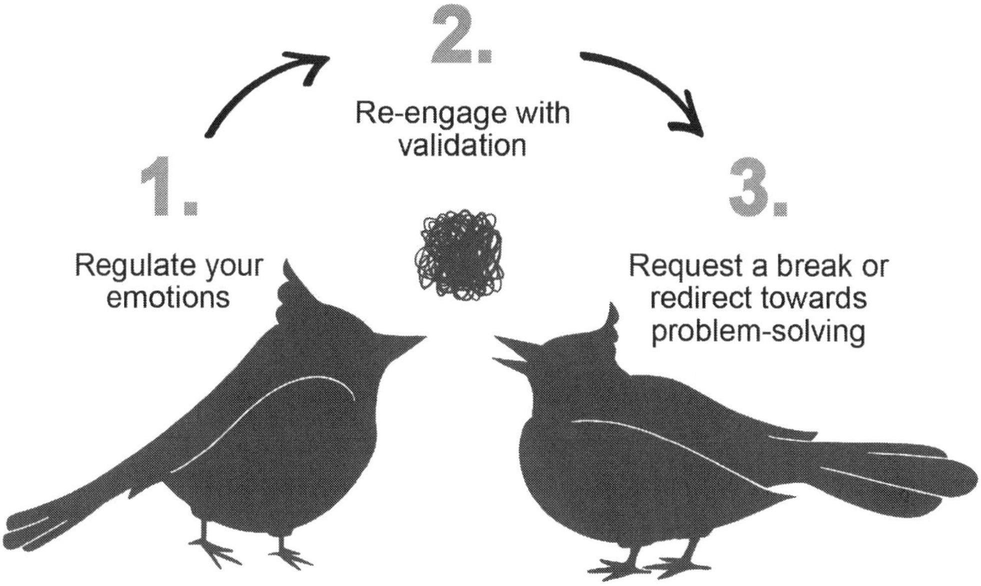
2.
Re-engage with validation
1.
Regulate your emotions
3.
Request a break or redirect towards problem-solving

1. If either of you is feeling reactive, communicate the need to pause so you can self-regulate or co-regulate using tools presented in Chapter 3.

2. As you begin to feel more regulated, re-engage by validating each other. This will help to de-escalate the tension by helping both partners feel heard and understood. Remember, validation is not agreement. It is the ability to recognize someone else's experience, even if your experience is different. To review tips on validation, you can revisit the section on page 107.

3. Once both partners feel validated, move towards problem-solving as members of the same team. How can the two of you work together to solve a problem that is inhibiting your ability to run a business together successfully?

4. If either of you is having trouble regulating, it may be a good idea to request a break and revisit the conversation at a later time. Make sure to agree upon the later time and follow through with it so the problem does not remain unresolved.

Approaching your relationship as a business partnership is suggested as a temporary coping strategy to help you meet the demands of the fourth trimester and navigate challenges more successfully as you settle into your new normal. As things begin to fall into place, you can adapt your weekly meetings to something that feels more natural and warm to you. However, if this strategy does not resonate for you, and you are experiencing distress related to division of labor, it may be a good idea to enlist the help of a couple's therapist who specializes in providing support to new parents or couples with small children.

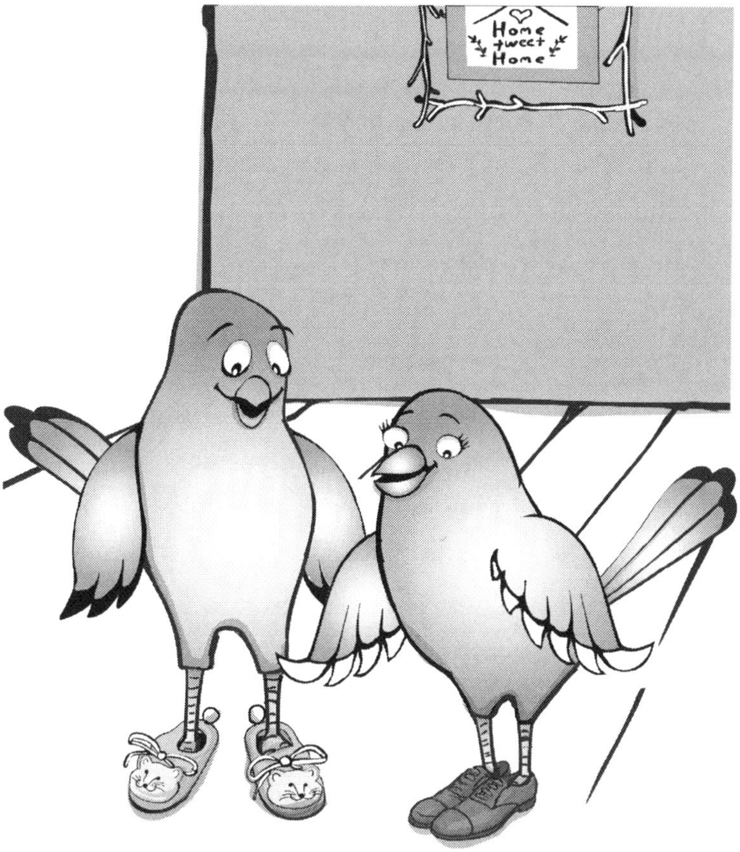
Home
tweet
Home

Regardless of how you choose to manage division of labor issues, I encourage you to make it a habit to step into each other's shoes. This will help you both recognize and appreciate the different ways in which each of you contributes to your family. This may also allow you both to be more open to listening and exploring new ways of supporting one another—imperfectly, but with progress.

Resentment and Loneliness

Mothers are often the primary parent, and these busy moms express a myriad of feelings when they come in to see me in the first year postpartum for individual or couples therapy. Two feelings that are identified frequently are resentment and loneliness. These feelings are sometimes attributed to experiencing drastic changes in their lives, compounded by the fact that mothers don't perceive their partner to experience changes to the same degree. Mothers in my practice describe feelings of resentment towards their partner for the simple fact that they feel tied down to the responsibility of breastfeeding and caring for their baby, while their partner seems to enjoy more freedom to continue living life the way they did before the baby arrived. They also express feeling lonely because they don't believe their partner fully understands or appreciates their difficult reality.

From the perception and experience of these mothers, their partner enjoys the freedom of having time away from the baby and parenting responsibilities because they go to work, going out as they please, engaging in a social life, continuing hobbies and interests such as sports, working out, or gaming, not carrying the mental load, and sleeping soundly without the pressure of having to respond to their baby's needs at night. Simultaneously, these mothers experience a loss of control in their own lives as they feel the burden of responsibilities as the primary parent, recognize their inability to enjoy the same freedoms as their partners, and experience challenges as their body continues to recover and change.

In couple's therapy, when I hear a mother describe these sentiments, I usually hear her partner respond in one of four ways: defend, deny, dismiss, or offer solutions. With any of these responses, the mother feels unseen and unheard. Unfortunately, defending yourself or denying her reality only makes her feel more resentful and alone. As the supportive partner, the best thing you can do is:

1. Avoid personalizing what she is sharing
2. Acknowledge her reality without "ifs" and "buts"
3. Validate her feelings sincerely
4. Ask her how you can support her better so she feels less resentful and alone

You can review the section on validation in the previous chapter to look at examples and remind yourself about what it is and how to offer it appropriately. Be sure to review other communication guidelines as well to help you remain present, responsive, and non-defensive if you are met with a harsh start-up or a criticism.

If you are the primary parent, reflect on how you may have communicated feelings of resentment or loneliness to your partner in the past, if at all. If your partner did not respond well, it could be possible they felt blamed for your feelings. While you may very well blame them for how you feel, unfortunately, using blaming language with your partner will not make you feel any more heard, understood, or supported. I invite you to also review the previous chapter to remind yourself about the guidelines I provided for effective communication.

As discussed earlier, practice explaining your concerns, sharing your feelings, and expressing your needs in a manner that makes it possible for your partner to listen and respond as you would hope for them to. You are more likely to receive a validating or reassuring response from them by using respectful communication. That being said, I am aware how difficult respectful communication can be when you are sleep deprived, frustrated, or feeling low. Thus, I suggest reflecting ahead of time on how (and when) you would like to approach your partner about your feelings.

Sleep deprivation reduces your window of tolerance significantly, making you more stressed, reactive, emotional, and dysregulated. Therefore, prioritizing your sleep is crucial. I emphasized this in Chapter 1 as part of meeting your physiological needs and provided tips on page 28. Avoiding sensitive topics if you are sleep deprived is equally important to remember.

In the empty talk bubble below, script out how you might start a conversation with your partner about feelings such as resentment and loneliness. For example, you may write something like:

"I'm sorry for lashing out last night about you going out for golf earlier in the day. I took some time to reflect this morning, and I realized I have been carrying resentment inside of me. The resentment is triggered every weekend when I see you go out for golf with your brother. I am happy you get the break you need—and I also know how important it is for you to continue playing golf on the weekends. Still, a part of me feels sad and frustrated for not being able to step out of the house and do the things I enjoy, like you do. I think I will feel less resentful if I can confidently leave the house knowing I can rely on you to care for Ava without needing my help. So here's an idea...how about on Friday evening I step out for a bit and give you the opportunity to spend time alone with Ava? This will also give me the chance to practice relying on you without worrying."

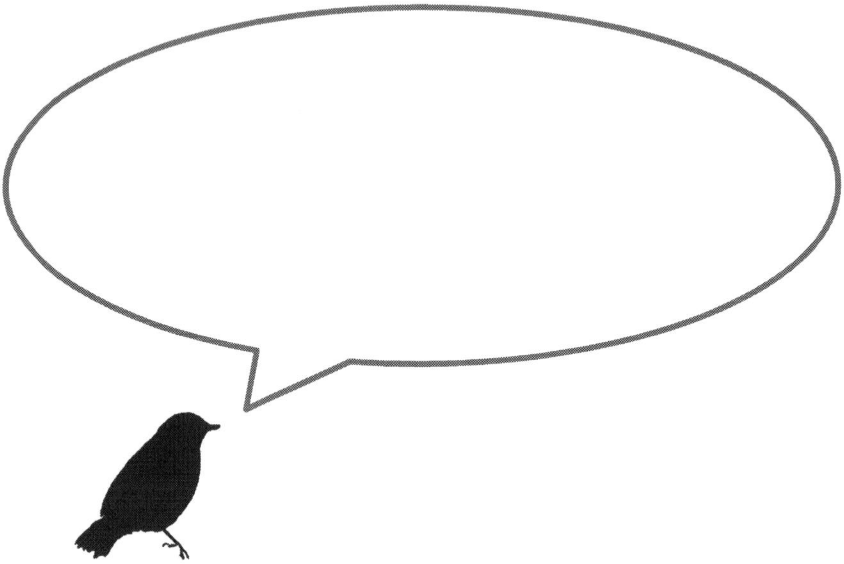

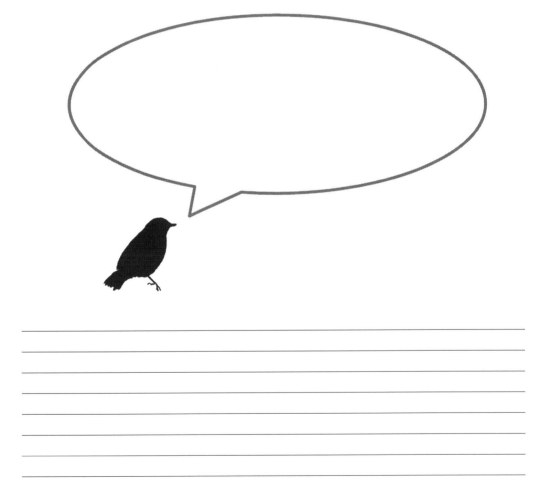

Different Parenting Styles

Amy and Neil met six years ago through friends and have been living together ever since Amy became pregnant with their child. They share a blended family of four children, three of whom are from previous marriages. Amy has an 11-year-old daughter from her first marriage, and Neil has an eight-year-old son and a nine-year-old daughter from his first marriage. Together, they have a son who is now three years old.

Since they both shared equal custody of their older children with their exes, the couple had all their children staying with them every alternating week. Soon after moving in with Neil, before their son was born, Amy started to feel concerned about the way he parented his children. She observed his interactions with them and how they would push boundaries and disrespect him.

Amy started to notice some changes in her daughter, who had also started pushing boundaries like her stepchildren. Amy, who grew up with strong boundaries in her household, continued to maintain boundaries firmly with her daughter and followed through with consequences consistently. In spite of her concerns, Amy avoided interfering with Neil's style of parenting his children and maintained her focus on parenting her daughter.

When the couple's son, James, was born three years ago, Amy experienced postpartum anxiety, which exacerbated over the years. She believed Neil's style of parenting was the reason her anxiety was not lessening. Despite Amy's continued efforts to maintain boundaries with their son, Neil would not uphold these boundaries in the same manner. For example, whenever James asked for more screen time, Neil would oblige despite Amy's objections. She blamed Neil for confusing James with conflicting messages by not supporting her parenting style. She believed her way of parenting was better. "Look at how disrespectful your children are with you and how they push you around! I don't want James to be that way with us when he is older. I can already see him behaving disrespectfully like his siblings. The fact that this doesn't bother you is very concerning."

Amy also expected Neil to enforce the boundaries she deemed necessary for their child's physical and mental development since she was the parent who was primarily involved in raising James. On the other hand, Neil argued their son was still quite young, and Amy was too strict with him. He also felt frustrated with how Amy dismissed his style of parenting and felt tired of being blamed for anything that went wrong when James was in Amy's care. "Any time he doesn't listen to her, she starts accusing me of spoiling him. She takes out all her frustration on me like it's my fault he's not listening. For God's sake, he's a kid! We both know kids don't listen easily at this age!" Neil exclaimed as he looked at Amy with frustration.

Amy felt resentful because the conflicting parenting styles threw off daily routines for their son, which not only increased Amy's stress and anxiety, but it also interfered with the couple's interactions with their older children. She also felt angry and exhausted because she found Neil's style of parenting counterproductive to her hard work as a parent. All of this led to tension and strain in the couple's relationship; they couldn't seem to agree on whose parenting style was better. The couple began to grow apart as the conflict continued in their relationship. James tested boundaries and experienced meltdowns almost daily. This contributed to feelings of anger, exhaustion, and resentment between both partners.

As demonstrated by Amy and Neil's story, differences in parenting styles can create tension and conflict in a couple's relationship. Parenting styles can become apparent shortly after birth when beliefs around breastfeeding, bottle feeding, or formula feeding are in conflict between the new parents. For example, one partner might feel adamant about their baby receiving breast milk, whereas the other might feel strongly about adequate nutrition, regardless of the type of milk. Other examples of differences which may show up as early as the first few days or weeks after birth are that of co-sleeping, implementing routines, and involvement of family members. As the baby grows into a toddler, differences in parenting can relate to the child's development, nutrition, discipline, boundaries, consequences, religion, education, language, and socialization.

Whatever the issue, the different ways of parenting can give rise to tension in the relationship, which can spill into the couple's interactions with each other. When this tension persists for an extended time with no resolve, negative communication cycles can develop involving critical, blaming, and defensive behaviors. Such interactions can lead to feelings of anger, irritability, impatience, and helplessness between the co-parents, chipping away at the emotional connection that was once shared between the two partners.

When a couple comes in to see me describing their disagreements on parenting, one of the things I find beneficial is to help them explore and understand their partner's style of parenting from a place of curiosity. I encourage them to ask questions respectfully and non-judgmentally to help them develop compassion and a new perspective instead of remaining entrenched in their positions on parenting. I also help them reflect on what is driving each person's need to maintain their way of parenting so strongly.

Sometimes, upon reflection, clients realize they were standing their ground for no other reason than their desire to feel heard and respected! When couples engage in this new process of approaching their differences in parenting, both partners begin to feel heard, understood, and respected. As a result, they begin to feel more open to the idea of evaluating their parenting styles.

As a couple assesses their parenting approach with newfound insight, conscious awareness, and a fresh perspective, it creates an opportunity for them to value each other's parenting, while honoring or modifying their own. It also provides opportunities to negotiate and reach common ground. To help you discover ways to explore your differences on parenting, I have listed four areas of discussion below. You can reflect on the questions on your own, or together as a couple.

1. **Explore what both of you learned about parenting from your upbringing.** In what ways do you parent your children similarly, or differently, than your parents? What changes would you like to make as you are consciously evaluating your parenting? If no change is desired, why is it important for you to maintain your approach to parenting?
2. **Recognize the values which influence your parenting decisions.** Where are these values coming from? What are some values that are common between the two of you? What are some values that are different? Which values are in conflict and causing tension in your relationship? How important is it for you to maintain the values that are in conflict? How can you negotiate these values to find harmony in your relationship? Which values would you like to consciously practice, modify or replace to change your approach to parenting?
3. **Identify expectations of yourself and your partner as a co-parenting team, and as a parent to your child(ren).** Where are these expectations coming from and how are they influencing your parenting? How are they impacting

your child(ren) and your co-parenting relationship? Which expectations need to be managed?

4. **Identify expectations each of you has of your child(ren).** Where are these expectations coming from and how are they influencing your parenting? How are they impacting your child(ren)? Are there any conflicting expectations of your child(ren) between you and your partner? How is this difference in expectations impacting your child(ren) and your co-parenting relationship? Which expectations need to be managed?

Ultimately, what I like to remind couples is the importance of being a co-parenting team. To be a team does not mean two people need to be identical in their parenting style. What it means is two people need to work together to respectfully negotiate and agree on how they would like to parent their children. If you are divided in a tug of war between who is right and who is wrong, it is unlikely to establish a strong co-parenting team. However, you can create a strong partnership if you learn to work together compassionately, bring out each other's strengths as parents, support each other where one of you may be struggling as a parent, be open to learning from your mistakes, compromise for the good of the team, be flexible enough in your parenting to create space for your partner's style of parenting, and display mutual respect.

Among the couples who come to see me describing tension in their relationship due to differences in parenting, I sometimes find one or both partners walking through the journey of parenthood without conscious awareness. This can be harmful if a parent carries on negative or toxic generational cycles by automatically repeating particular behaviors or communication patterns which they learned from their own parents. If this resonates with you, I encourage you to learn how to parent more consciously. In other words, consider making parenting choices based on increased self-awareness, present-day research, and following the guidance of experts in the field, such as child psychologists. Child psychologists are trained in the study of child development, and they provide recommendations to parents based on clinical evaluations and evidence-based research. Breaking harmful generational cycles may also involve working with a therapist to heal your inner child and learn to parent your children how you would have liked to be parented. I have provided resources on topics related to parenting and inner-child healing in Chapter 6.

Becoming conscious of your parenting style and recognizing your mistakes can be a difficult thing to face. As someone who is continuously learning to heal and grow in order to be a better parent to my children, I feel deep compassion and respect for the parents I work with who have the courage to break unhealthy generational patterns of parenting. Some of these parents experience a painful yet powerful process of recognizing and healing the wounds of their inner child while learning to respond in new ways to their children. Through this process, parents create a more safe and secure environment for their children by consistently practicing healthier, more responsive, and developmentally nurturing ways of parenting.

Before I end this section, I want to gently remind you that secure attachment is developed in the journey of a relationship through repeated and *consistent* interactions that establish feelings of trust, safety, and security. Therefore, raising securely attached children is a life-long process. A secure attachment cannot be broken in an instance—unless a child experiences trauma, such as any kind of abuse or form of neglect. This means that a minor mistake as a parent does not determine the outcome of your child's relationship or attachment with you. If you make a mistake, the most important thing to remember is to repair and restore the trust and safety your child normally feels in their relationship with you.

For example, imagine a scenario where you cooked a fresh meal for your two-year-old toddler. After several failed attempts of trying to get them to eat their dinner, your toddler immediately throws the food to the ground. You are six months pregnant with your second child, physically tired, and emotionally drained from a long day of managing tantrums. In a moment of rage, you scream at them, leaving your toddler feeling terrified and crying hysterically. You immediately regret screaming and feel guilty, but you are too upset to comfort them. You ask your partner to step into the kitchen and comfort your child as you walk to a different room to regulate yourself.

You return to your toddler five minutes later, take them in your arms, and explain to them what happened in a gentle manner and using age-appropriate language. You take responsibility for reacting poorly to feelings of exhaustion and anger so your toddler is not left assuming that you screamed at them because of who they are. Developmentally, children are unable to understand abstract concepts. They view the world through a simplistic, black or white lens: "I am good" or "I am bad"; "Mommy loves me" or "Mommy does not love me"; "my feelings matter" or "my feelings don't matter." This is why it is important to explain to your child what happened so they can differentiate that you disapprove of their behavior, not them.

To make amends, you can take ownership and apologize for your behavior, validate your child's feelings, and establish a boundary so they understand how to communicate with you next time. For example, you can say in a comforting tone, *"I am so sorry for how Mommy (or Daddy) reacted. It wasn't a nice way to express my frustration, and I scared you. If I feel frustrated again, I will take deep breaths to keep myself calm. And if you don't feel like eating the meal I give you, instead of throwing food on the ground, you can tell me, 'I am full' or 'I don't want this.'"*

If your child is too young to understand what you are saying, you can use physical comfort as a way to help regulate your child and reestablish safety for them. An example of this is hugging your child as you gently rock them for a few minutes. You can also tell them something simple to help them make sense of their experience and feel safe again, *"Mommy (or Daddy) screamed and Ollie got scared? I am so sorry. I love you so much!"*

When ruptures are repaired quickly and consistently in the manner I have outlined, a child comes to know their parents as trustworthy, reliable, consistent, and safe people to be around. They learn to predict that their parents will be there for them to help regulate, comfort, and make amends if there is a rupture in the connection, which leads to a more securely attached parent-child relationship.

Effects of the Pandemic

As I write this book, we are in the third year of the COVID-19 pandemic, which continues to have a significant impact on relationships around the world. Couples have found themselves in new, unchartered territory: They are together 24/7, working from home, juggling childcare, homeschooling, and household duties, managing the uncertainties and logistical nightmares that come with any family member displaying "symptoms," isolating, facing financial stressors and/or loss of employment, and parenting—all at the same time! The pandemic has also given rise to postpartum mood disturbances among women who have had children during this time (Vigod et al., 2021).

With less time spent apart, more responsibilities, fewer opportunities to take a break or engage in one's interests and hobbies, inability to socialize with family and friends, lack of access to medical care and childcare, and increased feelings of uncertainty, confusion, anxiety, stress, and depression, couples with small children have faced a myriad of unique challenges. With the stressors of the pandemic burdening a couple's relationship, those who have sought therapy with me during 2020-2022 have reported varying levels of distress and suffering.

As the pandemic continues to impact the postpartum population I work with in Ontario, more couples have reported increased tension and conflict, feeling unfulfilled, and losing the connection they once shared. I have heard these couples describe themselves and their relationship in the following ways:

- *"We are just roommates."*
- *"We no longer do things as a couple even though we are around each other 24/7."*
- *"I am wiped out between working and watching the kids. By the end of the day, I just want to go into my separate corner and be alone."*
- *"There has been tension between us because we have different tolerance levels around COVID, and we disagree on what is safe for us and our children."*
- *"We are cohabitants."*
- *"We are quick to attack each other."*
- *"It is hard for us to connect or do things together when there is nowhere to go."*
- *"We have become impatient with each other."*
- *"We try to keep it together in front of our co-workers and our kids while we work from home, but we take out our frustrations on each other."*

While it is true some couples have disconnected or broken up during the pandemic, there are also couples who have come together and built a stronger connection. These couples have developed good coping skills to manage stressors and figured out ways to adjust to a new normal. Spending time together in ways that was not possible before the pandemic has allowed these couples to get to know each other better, problem-solve together, provide support to each other, and learn to work as a team.

Similarly, if you also want to learn how to make a better team, here are five ways you can develop a strong partnership during challenging times:

1. **Communicate**: Prioritize a few minutes each week to sit together and evaluate what is working and what is not working in terms of your relationship, childcare, schedules, work, house chores, and so forth. During this time, make sure to check in with each other's needs by asking your partner how you can be more helpful and supportive the following week. Practice flexibility, adapt to changing circumstances, and discuss ways in which you can work together to balance your needs, your partner's needs, and your children's needs.

2. **Share responsibility**: Work together as a team to assign and share tasks by creating an exhaustive list of items you both have on your plates. This includes but is not limited to: managing work schedules, childcare (meals, naps, baths, bed times, appointments), cooking, cleaning, taking the garbage out, doing groceries, and managing family activities. Do the best you can to support each other in meeting your demands where neither of you has too much on your plate at any given time. Once again, remain flexible and open to changing roles and responsibilities as you continue to communicate about what is working and what is not working.

3. **Set boundaries**: Initiate ways in which you can create a healthy work-life balance, especially if you are still working from home. If it is helpful, establish routines and/or schedules which you both can agree upon or feel satisfied with. As you work towards establishing a routine, here are a few boundaries to consider for yourself: What time will you sleep and what time will you start your day? What time will you clock in to work? When will you eat lunch? What time will you end work? Which days will you exercise or fulfill an interest of yours? When will you spend time with the kids? When will you

spend time with your partner? At what point will you set your phone and/or laptop aside to give your family undivided attention?

4. **Schedule time for yourself**: Being together all the time may work well for some couples, but for many, it can test the relationship in ways mentioned earlier. For some people, it is pivotal to their mental health to spend some time alone every day or every week. This can be especially true for the parent who is primarily responsible for childcare because they give so much of their physical, mental, and emotional energy into the parent-child relationship. At some point in their day, they need time to regain their energy through a self-fulfilling activity, such as resting in a quiet place, reading a book, watching a show, engaging in a hobby, enjoying a cup of tea, or connecting with a loved one. If this resonates for you, enlist your partner's support in carving out daily or weekly personal time. If this sounds like your partner, encourage them to prioritize personal time.

5. **Schedule time for each other**: As important as it can be to schedule time for yourself, it is equally important to spend time with your partner—without children! To maintain a strong connection, schedule quality time for your relationship. It can range from a few minutes spent together every day, to a couple of hours every week, to a regular day each month. How much time you need to spend together to maintain a good connection depends on every couple and can differ between two people. Therefore, make a concerted effort to satisfy both partners' needs. Finally, be mindful that the *quality* of time you spend together matters more in building and maintaining connection than spending a large amount of time together.

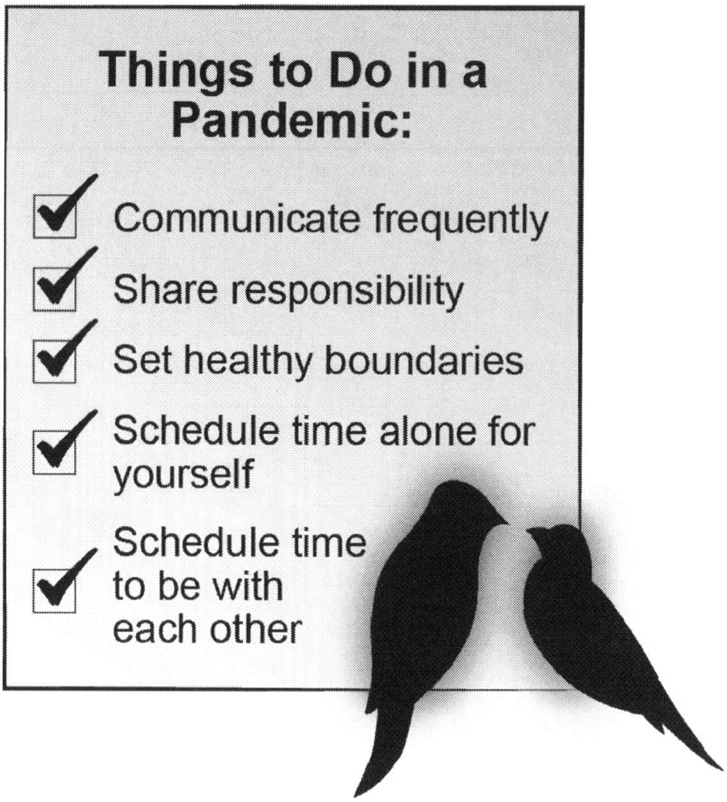
Things to Do in a Pandemic:
Communicate frequently
Share responsibility
Set healthy boundaries
Schedule time alone for yourself
Schedule time to be with each other

These suggestions can be useful for all couples trying to cope with the stressors of the pandemic, regardless of whether they have children or not. If you are reading this after the pandemic has subsided, this information also applies to couples who may be dealing with chronic illness, financial distress, a natural disaster, or some other circumstance that requires they spend a great deal of time together in the home. Working as a team is an integral part of navigating difficult times in your life. While adversity can pull you apart, it can also create opportunities for you to become stronger together. Which couple will you be?

Conflicting Values

Values are the fundamental principles or set of beliefs that guide your life and motivate your daily actions, consciously or unconsciously. They are the spoken or unspoken messages you grew up with. Values can be intrinsic or extrinsic, meaning they can come from within or be placed upon you by an external source, such as family, religion, culture, and society. For example, if your parents repeatedly told you the importance of working hard in life when you were a child, or they demonstrated the importance of hard work through their actions and the way they lived their life, you may grow up to become a hardworking person. This is because the value of hard work was ingrained in you. Consciously, or unconsciously, it may have become a fundamental principle in your life.

There are many different types of values a person can uphold in their life. Figure 14 displays a non-exhaustive list of individual, relationship, and family values.

Figure 14

Examples of different types of values

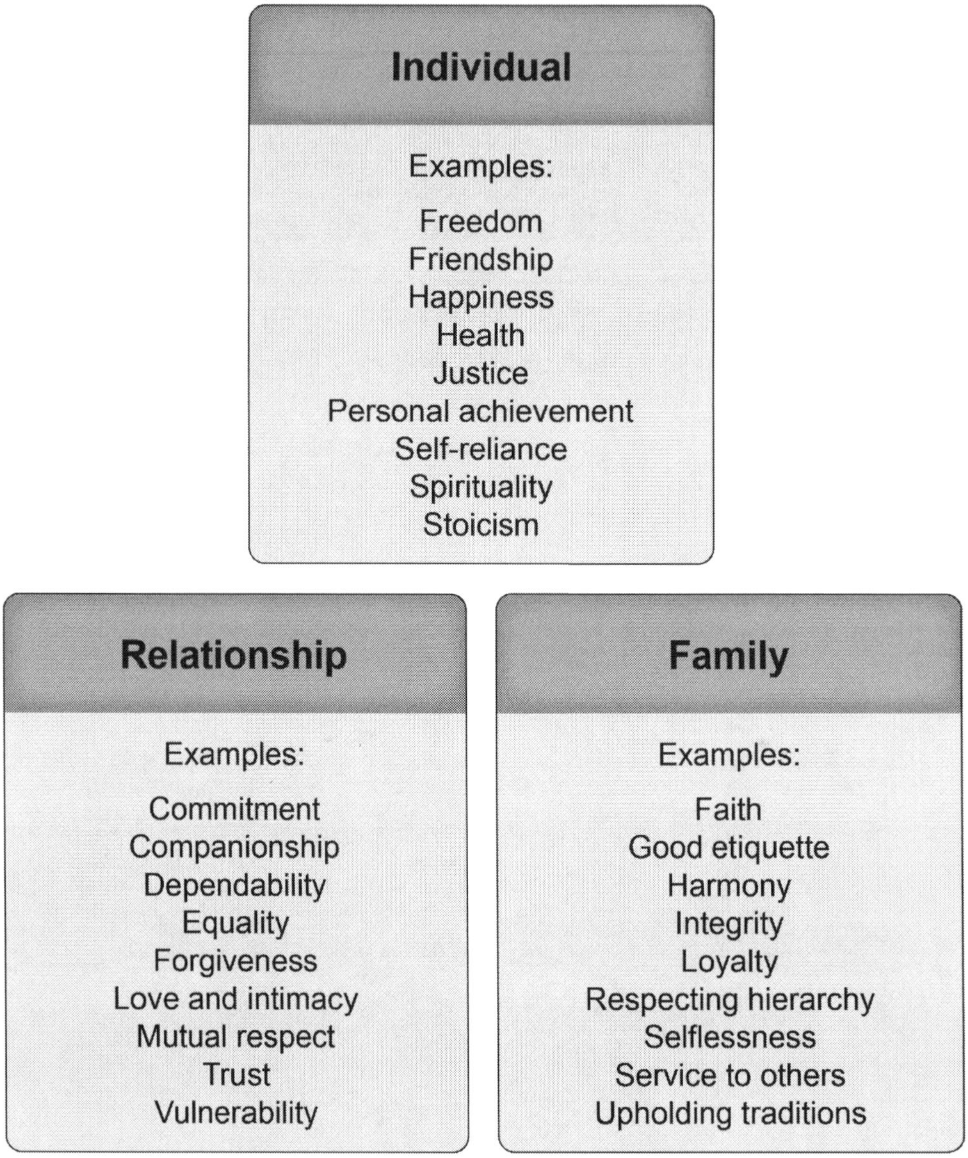
Individual
Examples:
Freedom
Friendship
Happiness
Health
Justice
Personal achievement
Self-reliance
Spirituality
Stoicism
Relationship
Examples:
Commitment
Companionship
Dependability
Equality
Forgiveness
Love and intimacy
Mutual respect
Trust
Vulnerability
Family
Examples:
Faith
Good etiquette
Harmony
Integrity
Loyalty
Respecting hierarchy
Selflessness
Service to others
Upholding traditions

In a relationship, each person brings their own set of values. Some values can be mutually shared, and others can be different. Tension can surface when two people's values are in direct conflict with each other. The following is an example of conflicting values in a couple's relationship.

Tanya and Caleb shared a loving marital relationship where they both understood each other and managed their differences well. However, since the birth of their daughter 15 months ago, their difference in certain values created tension in their relationship. They were not able to see eye to eye nor were they able to accept the difference because each spouse felt strongly about their values.

Tanya wanted her husband to be more proactive in helping her raise their daughter. However, Caleb struggled to tune out the demands of work to prioritize spending more time with their daughter. Tanya found this upsetting because she believed family should be her husband's top priority. She grew up with parents who were equally involved in her life, and she shared a special bond with her father. Tanya wanted her daughter to have the same bond with Caleb. She feared that Caleb would not be able to have a good relationship with their daughter unless he prioritized her from a young age.

Caleb, who deeply loved his wife and daughter, felt conflicted because financial success was something he strongly believed should be achieved from a young age. It was important to Caleb to create a secure and stable life for himself and his family. He believed if he worked hard and achieved financial success, he would be able to enjoy the fruits of his labor later in life and spend ample time with his family.

Tanya and Caleb's case exemplifies how values can come into conflict and put a strain on a couple's relationship, especially after having a baby. Sometimes, couples are not aware of this conflict until they attend therapy to explore their concerns. If you are experiencing ongoing tension, disagreements, or disconnection in your relationship without an apparent reason, it might be worthwhile to explore both your value systems to determine if there are any conflicting values between the two of you. You can start by creating separate lists of what each of you identifies as your set of values. As a reminder, values are the set of principles, fundamentals, or beliefs you live by. Figure 14 can guide this process by helping you brainstorm. After you and your partner have identified your values, reflect on which values you mutually share and which ones are different.

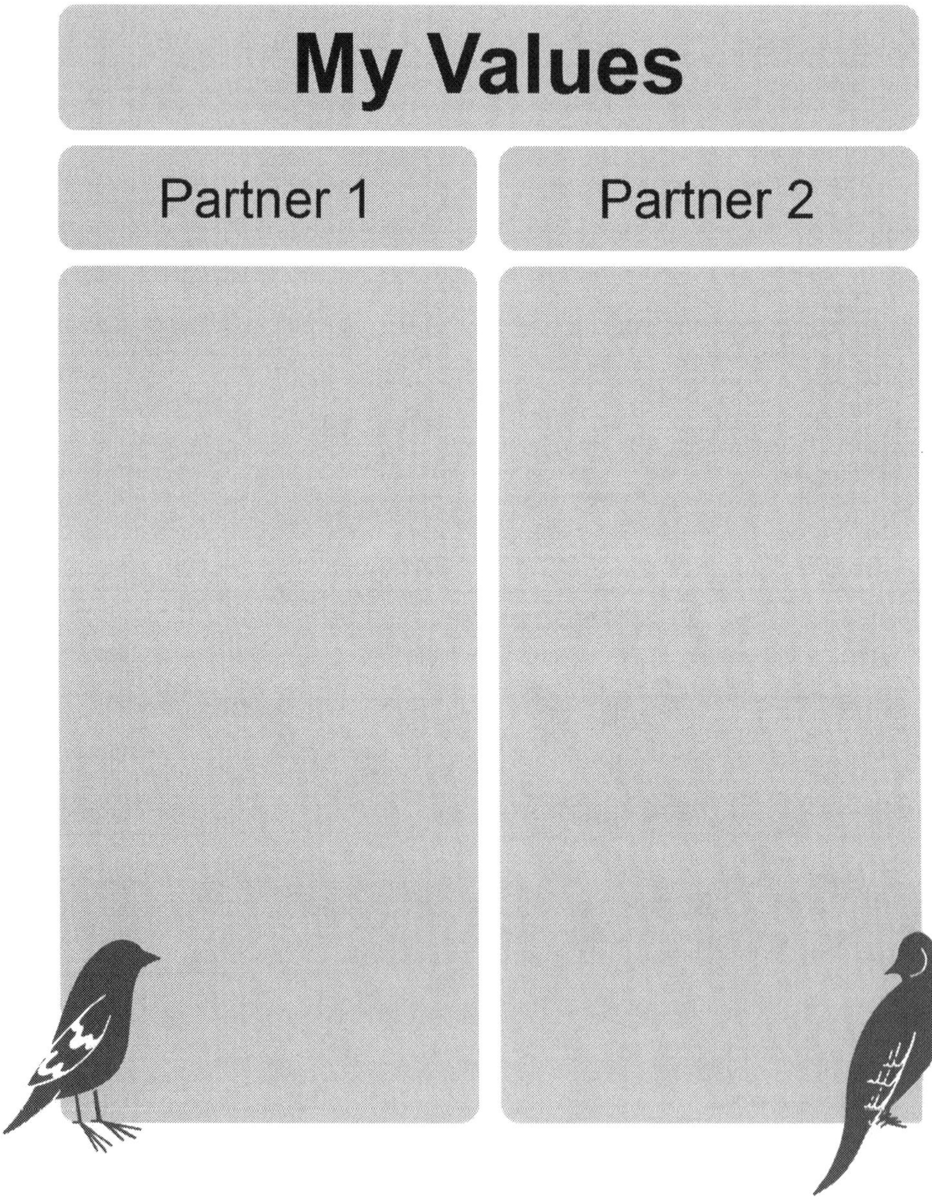
My Values
Partner 1
Partner 2

Doing this exercise will help you determine if there are any conflicting values which may be contributing to the disagreements or tension in your relationship. It will also help you reevaluate which values you'd like to continue practicing in your life and which you'd like to replace. In Caleb's case, he might realize that while financial success is important to him, having strong family connections is also important; therefore, he might make a conscious decision to be more involved in his daughter's life.

It is vitally important to mention that values are not fixed. They can change and evolve over time. For example, if you were someone who once valued adventure and spontaneity, you may come to value comfort and stability after having your first child. It is also normal for one value, or a set of values, to become more relevant than others during a certain time of your life. For example, parenting values might become more relevant in your life when you have small children and become less relevant as your children grow into adults.

Finally, it is also possible for one or both people in a relationship to experience a shift in their values, such that it causes friction between them. If the couple is able to remain constant in their foundational values, that is, values that pertain to deal-breakers, then changes in other values can be manageable. A deal-breaker is any value, quality, or behavior of your partner which you disagree with on a fundamental level and are unable to resolve or compromise. Deal-breakers can be related to religion, monogamy, trust, commitment, marriage, where you live, the decision to have children and/or how many, how you parent the children, career, politics, addictions, abuse, and so on.

Each couple has their unique foundational values because what is a deal-breaker in your relationship might not be a deal-breaker in another couple's relationship; therefore, it is not helpful to compare your relationship with others. With conscious awareness, vulnerable communication, openness, flexibility, compromise, and acceptance, it is possible for a couple to live in harmony even when they have differing values.

Sex and Intimacy

During pregnancy, it is normal for a woman's sexual desire and functioning to decrease (Ninivaggio et al., 2017; Bartellas et al., 2000). Partners also experience changes in their sexual desire, though it behaves differently between men and women in pregnancy. In one study, both men and women experienced lower sexual desire during pregnancy; however, men's desire remained consistently higher than their female partner's (Fernández-Carrasco et al., 2020).

It is also common for postpartum couples to experience a negative impact on their sex life due to sexual dissatisfaction, low desire, and increased sexual distress (Schwenck et al., 2020). In a study examining the risk factors involved in postpartum sexual dysfunction among mothers (Gutzeit et al., 2020), the authors cite findings where anywhere from 41 percent to as many as 83 percent of women have been found to experience sexual dysfunction 2-3 months after birth (Barrett et al., 2000; Signorello et al., 2001) and up to 64 percent of mothers at 6 months after birth (McDonald et al., 2017).

Based on my professional experience, the following is a list of factors that can adversely influence a mother's sexuality, which in turn, impacts the physical and sexual intimacy between her and her partner:

- Sleep deprivation
- Lack of time and energy
- Baby's physical needs
- Baby's medical needs
- Hormonal imbalance
- Physical recovery and pain
- Birth trauma

- Feeling touched out
- Body image issues
- Poor mental health
- Relationship dissatisfaction
- Burnout

Mothers are not the only ones who experience changes in their sexuality. Fathers also experience highs and lows in sexual functioning after the birth of their child, with fatigue, stress, and time constraints being the main reasons for their low desire in the first three months postpartum (Van Anders, 2013). With the challenges that new parents face in the first year after birth, it's understandable why many of them report decreased intimacy. Regardless of how frequently you engaged in intimate acts before your little one arrived, sex may be the farthest thing from your mind for some time after birth, especially if you're the birthing parent who is also the primary caregiver to your child. Among couples who welcome more children into their family, low intimacy may be prevalent for a few years.

Based on my observations of parents with small children who come to me for couple's therapy, some of them carry unrealistic expectations around sexual intimacy. These couples make comparisons between what their sex life looked like before they became parents versus after they became parents. I believe this comparison is unfair considering the drastic changes these couples have experienced since becoming parents. Some couples also compare themselves to other parents who they perceive as enjoying a healthier sex life.

If you and/or your partner make similar comparisons, please know that while sex is a healthy expression of love, intimacy, and connection in a couple's relationship, it is not the only form of expression. Additionally, how often you and your partner engage in sexual intimacy is personal to your relationship; it is not healthy emotionally or mentally to compare your sex life to another couple.

One factor which I would like to highlight as a strong influencer of a couple's physical and sexual intimacy is their emotional connection. This is something I have learned through my clinical observations. I have found that while couples may be able to engage in the physical act of sex regardless of their connection, their *desire* for sex and intimacy is less likely to be present without emotional connection. This seems especially true among the women I support in therapy.

A conversation is warranted between you and your partner if either of you feels unsettled by the quality of your physical and/or sexual intimacy. With mutual respect and vulnerability by both partners, a meaningful conversation can resolve misunderstandings, bring clarity, repair damage, increase compassion, and deepen emotional connection. Even if feelings of desire do not increase as an outcome of this conversation, the partner who has low or no sexual desire might feel more inclined to address and improve intimacy issues for the health of the relationship.

A conversation can also resolve any issues which could be inhibiting emotional, physical, and sexual intimacy in a relationship. For example, imbalance of needs, resentment, or unfair division of labor could all be reasons for weakened emotional connection between two partners, adversely impacting their physical and sexual intimacy. Therefore, a respectful conversation where these issues are identified, explored, and addressed can lead to increased intimacy in all areas of the relationship.

Let's take a look at the dialogue between Rebecca and Derek, a married couple with an 11-month-old daughter:

Derek:
"I noticed how little you want to be with me nowadays and how often you push me away when I try to be intimate with you. I've been feeling confused for a while, and now I am starting to feel resentful."

Rachel:
"What you're saying sounds important, and I want to make sure I give you my undivided attention. Right now, I am feeling a bit overwhelmed. Daisy is teething and is having a rough day today. I want to get her dinner ready so she can go to bed on time. How about we talk tonight once she's asleep?"

Derek:
"Sounds good. I can put Daisy to sleep after dinner so you can get some rest before we talk."

Later that night...

Rachel:
"You had some concerns about us not having sex?"

Derek:
"Yes, we used to have sex once or twice a week before Daisy was born. Now, we hardly have it once in a month. And even so, I have this feeling you don't want to. I don't like forcing it on you but having sex and being intimate is important to me. I feel rejected. And I feel dirty when I am forcing this on you... I feel unwanted."

Rachel:
"I didn't realize you were feeling all those things."

Derek:
"I wasn't at first, but I am now. Daisy is almost a year old. I am starting to get worried about us. I worry if you still love me."

Rachel:
"I do love you. I'm just so exhausted from everything. I feel like we are either running around working, doing things around the house, or taking care of Daisy. When you and I talk, it's always about chores or Daisy. And we don't even talk, we argue most of the time."

Derek:
"I agree, we argue a lot. And we don't talk about anything fun anymore."

Rachel:
"We don't. And a lot of that is because of the pandemic, I think. We are with each other 24/7 and neither of us does much outside of the house anymore. I don't know what we are supposed to talk about when we have been around each other all day."

Derek:
"But it isn't just about the talking. I don't even think you want to hang out with me after Daisy is in bed. I would love to put on a show and watch it with you but any time I make the suggestion, I hear all the reasons why you can't watch it with me. And it would be nice if sometimes you initiated sex."

Rachel:
"I wish I could - I just feel too tired. And, frankly, I don't feel like having sex with someone who I have been arguing with all day. None of our arguments ever resolve and I feel frustrated inside. It's probably the same reason why I don't feel like watching a show or doing anything with you."

Derek:
"Okay so you're saying that you don't feel like having sex because you are tired from the day and frustrated with me?"

Rachel:
"I'm exhausted, yes. I'm not frustrated with you because I'm also at fault for arguing with you. I'm frustrated at the fact that we can't have a normal conversation anymore. The bickering makes me even more tired and nothing gets resolved."

Derek:
"I get it. You're exhausted and frustrated from all the arguing. And I think it's important for you to know I'm feeling alone and unwanted, and it's building up resentment inside of me."

In this dialogue, both Rachel and Derek have implemented effective communication tools to talk about a sensitive topic. They have demonstrated listening skills to understand each other better instead of interrupting, dismissing, or reacting. They have also demonstrated self-awareness, validation, compassion, and vulnerability. If the couple continues engaging in this dialogue, they can work together to identify the underlying problem causing their frequent arguments. They can also explore different ways Derek can offer more support to Rebecca so she feels less exhausted and more inclined to meet Derek's needs of spending time together and sexual intimacy.

If you are considering having a conversation with your partner to address issues around sex and intimacy, I recommend reviewing communication tools in Chapter 3.

Relationship Dissatisfaction

With so much happening in a couple's life after the birth of a tiny human, it is not uncommon for their relationship to experience challenges.

Sometimes old wounds are triggered, other times new wounds are created. Even among the couples who otherwise share a strong and secure partnership, feelings of tension and disconnection can be present for some time after their baby is born. In fact, research demonstrates how marital functioning declines after the birth of a couple's first child due to relationship dissatisfaction, poor conflict management, and negative patterns of communication (Doss et al., 2009). Given how inevitable it seems to be, it raises the question why couples are not prepared with tools ahead of time to support their relationship as it weathers the storm of those first few months after birth.

It is not necessarily an overnight shift that happens in a couple's relationship. It is usually a buildup over time of the day-to-day reality after the baby arrives. Two people who were romantic partners to each other also become co-parents of a child. The couple's needs are no longer the center of attention. The demands of taking care of a baby are high. Life as you knew it no longer exists. Before your baby was born, especially for the primary parent, you lived your life according to your own will. After your baby arrived, you experienced a dramatic shift in living your life according to your baby's fundamental needs.

As I spoke about earlier in this chapter, it is mothers who typically fall into the primary caregiver role, or they choose to be in that role. For new mothers, their life and most decisions they make revolve around their baby, such as how often will their baby need to be fed and at what intervals, when do they need a diaper change, a bath, or a nap, what time will they sleep at night and what time will they wake up, when do they need their next check-up with the doctor, what should go inside their diaper bag, how much milk needs to be pumped, how frequently, and how to balance this with breastfeeding, when will they need to start solids, and the list is endless! It is the day-to-day repetitive nature of responsibilities, tasks, and decisions that start to take a toll on a mother, and ultimately her relationship.

The parent who is in the supporting role may be doing their best to help in whatever capacity they can, or however much they are willing to. However, as time goes on,

- Priorities can shift
- Roles can evolve
- Responsibilities can pile up
- Expectations can be unfulfilled
- Needs can be unrecognized
- Conversations can become difficult

Furthermore, if the mother experiences a postpartum mood disturbance, such as anxiety and/or depression, it can become another source of distress in the couple's relationship. As explained in Chapter 1 of this book, it is important to recognize when you may be experiencing difficulties in managing your mood and emotions in the postpartum period and seek appropriate help to improve your mental health.

While these are a few ways a couple can experience dissatisfaction in their relationship after birth, there are also ways new parents can prevent dissatisfaction or reduce its occurrence. Based on his research on marital satisfaction among new parents (Shapiro et al., 2000), Gottman provides three tips which you can consciously implement with your partner after you welcome your baby:

1. **Be friends:** Maintain your pre-baby friendship during the transition to parenthood. Don't lose sight of who you were to each other before you became parents. Keep getting to know each other on an intimate level, as you would with a friend. Continue to acquaint yourself to each other's thoughts and feelings by:

- Asking questions, paying attention, and listening about each other's day
- Sharing about the ups and downs you experienced in other relationships, such as with friends, family members, or co-workers
- Celebrating joys and grieving sorrows together

2. **Listen and support:** Avoid letting the stressors of daily life build up inside of you. Continue to share your frustrations with each other as you would before the baby arrived. For example, was it a rough day at work? Was your baby being extra fussy? Did you forget to do something important? Use your stressful experiences as opportunities to be vulnerable with your partner and receive their comfort, support, and encouragement. This will help both of you feel connected, like you're "in it" together. If you are experiencing difficulty in communicating, connecting, or feeling safe with your partner, or if your partner seems emotionally unavailable or unresponsive to you, review the concepts, tools, and suggestions from Chapter 2 and Chapter 3 to navigate this issue effectively. For additional support, enlist the help of a therapist.

3. **Be gentle:** If something is upsetting you, be mindful of how you approach the conversation or disagreement. Saying something harshly will most likely elicit a defensive, blaming, withdrawing, or another reactive response from your partner. Furthermore, it will result in a break in your connection. Therefore, approach your partner with positive intentions and make an effort to engage in productive, meaningful conversations using the communication skills presented in this book. Remember, a gentle approach can build connection because it is more likely to create opportunities for vulnerability, understanding, compassion, problem-solving, and teamwork.

Compatibility

A challenging but important topic to discuss is the issue of compatibility. This can be a frightening or heartbreaking issue for new parents to consider. If you have been struggling with this, I want to sensitively step into this next section with you.

Working with new parents, I sometimes witness uncertainty among couples about whether they should continue their relationship. This uncertainty arises from a fear of incompatibility. Some couples worry they are growing apart because of the differences that are becoming more apparent as they take on new roles and responsibilities. These couples share the following doubts and concerns in therapy:

- Is it a good idea to stay together if we are so different?
- Are we ever going to get along again?
- Will we ever agree on how to parent and raise our child?
- Did we choose the wrong person to have a baby with?
- Are we compatible?

If this sounds like you, I would like to gently remind you that everything is new and different than what you've known before. Hence, it may require patience and time along with professional support and healthy coping strategies. Even if this is your second or third child together, it is still a new learning curve because being parents to one child is different from being parents to multiple children. Therefore, the issue might have less to do with your level of compatibility and more to do with your lack of adjustment. You may need more time to process and adjust to all the new things you are learning about yourself and each other as you simultaneously enter parenthood and a co-parenting relationship.

When I meet couples doubting their compatibility, I ask them about the reasons that brought them together in the first place. I ask them about how they met, what attracted them to each other, and what they liked, enjoyed, and valued about each other in the early stages of their relationship. I ask these questions to help couples remember all the reasons why they chose to be with each other and stay together before they had their children. Through this discussion, I often find the reasons that brought two people together are buried or forgotten under the strain of new roles and responsibilities.

If you are questioning your compatibility or having doubts about your relationship, it might be helpful to reflect on the reasons why you started dating each other and the reasons why you chose to commit to one another. It might also give you some hope to know that with time, many couples discover new ways of connecting, appreciating, and nurturing their relationship. The most important thing to remember is the challenges that come with raising small children and the strain they put on a couple's relationship are temporary. And it is possible to overcome these challenges with patience, compassion, forgiveness, and respect. In addition to this book, it may be beneficial for you to seek couple's therapy if you and your partner are experiencing dissatisfaction in your relationship.

Couples Who Are Incompatible

While the tools in this book can be helpful for all couples, this book is not designed for co-parenting couples who are no longer in a relationship. However, as a support, I wanted to outline a few ideas for couples who have decided they are not compatible and are choosing to co-parent outside of a committed relationship. These couples can do several things to make the transition from a romantic relationship to a co-parenting partnership less stressful. Here are a few suggestions:

1. Work with a therapist to help you manage potential differences in opinions in order to come to mutual agreements.
2. Establish ground rules around communication, visitation, vacations, holidays, schoolwork, and other important parenting

decisions. If there is high conflict with your co-parent, navigating this with a third party such as a family mediator can be very helpful.

3. Learn how to communicate your expectations of each other as co-parents in a way that is respectful. Have a tool for triggers, such as an emotion regulation technique (examples on page 91 and page 99) so you can stay present during difficult conversations.
4. Identify, communicate, and maintain your boundaries with yourself and your co-parent. It is important to communicate your boundaries in a clear and respectful manner in order to reduce conflict.
5. Learn conflict resolution tools, such as the one on page 144.
6. Attend parenting classes if need be.
7. Establish boundaries that protect the children instead of dragging them into conflicts you are working through.
8. Create a calendar that supports and respects each co-parent's schedule.
9. Focus on the well-being of your children, knowing and understanding that you may have different ideas about what is best for them.
10. Though you are no longer in a romantic relationship, it is important to still maintain a team mindset.
11. Extend flexibility when your co-parent may, on occasion, need to change the schedule due to work or personal reasons.
12. Review the communication tools outlined in Chapter 3; these apply to all healthy relationships, including a co-parenting partnership.
13. Make co-parenting decisions based on what is best for your child(ren), and not what is best for your needs.
14. Be mindful of how you speak about your co-parent around your child(ren) because it can impact their mental health and their relationship with both parents.
15. Do your best not to speak poorly of your co-parent with mutual friends or family members because it can increase negative perceptions and feelings towards your co-parent.

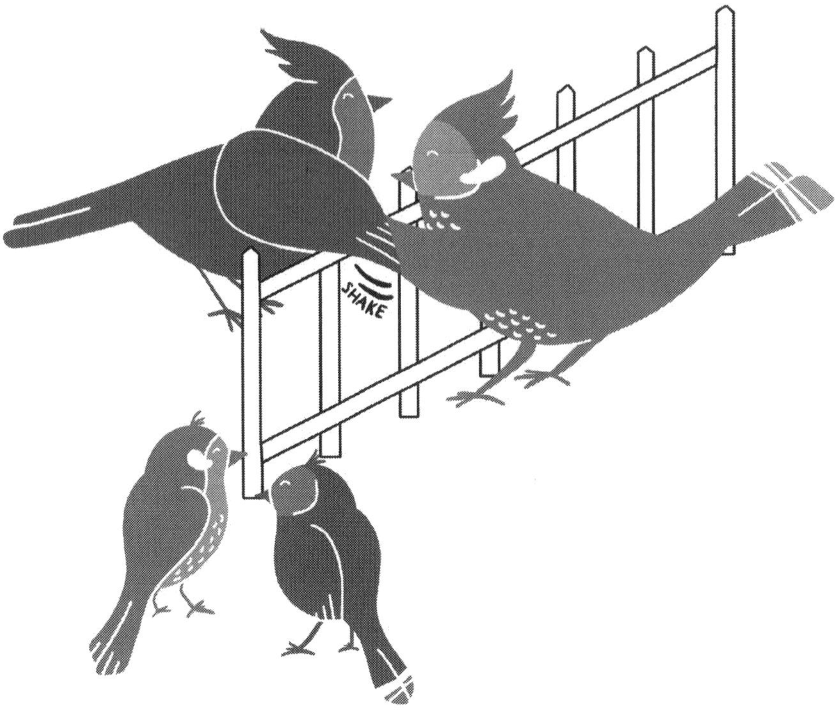
SHAKE

Along with the above suggestions, it is wise to invest time in reading books by experts on co-parenting strategies. I have suggested a few resources in Chapter 6.

Communication Breakdown

Couples can find themselves stuck in negative communication patterns as they face challenges involved in caring for a baby or raising small children. It isn't surprising, considering how parents can experience impatience and low tolerance with each other due to sleep deprivation, fatigue, and managing several roles and responsibilities. I find communication tends to suffer more when one or both partners have unfulfilled needs.

For example, a mother may experience disconnection from her partner if she feels unsupported for a prolonged period of time. As a result, she may push her partner away when they reach for physical affection. In this example, where the mother's need for support and her partner's need for affection are unsatisfied, both people may start engaging in maladaptive communication patterns. Maladaptive behaviors, such as criticizing, blaming, avoiding, hostility, passive aggression, contempt, and stonewalling prevent a couple's ability to successfully adapt and adjust to their circumstances. Such behaviors also interfere with their daily interactions and activities, ultimately wearing down their connection.

At a time when your relationship is under the strain of adjusting to raising a baby or children together, it becomes more necessary than ever before to engage in respectful, kind, and vulnerable forms of communication. The more you are able to communicate effectively, the more successfully you can navigate life together after birth.

Interestingly, if you are a mother, you are more likely to experience a decline in your marital satisfaction if your spouse interacts negatively with you (Shapiro et al., 2000). Conversely, when your spouse interacts fondly with you, you are more likely to experience greater marital satisfaction. These findings support the need for compassion in your communication, especially after the birth of your child. If you're a spouse reading this, now is a good time to take some notes!

That being said, communication occurs between two people, and both partners should be mindful of how they are interacting with each other. If you're the primary parent, I understand how difficult it can be to pay attention and think about how you are communicating if you are stretched thin and depleted of energy, tolerance, and patience. Becoming aware of your needs and communicating them, asking for help and support using effective communication tools, and applying self-care strategies from the next chapter may help you feel less depleted and more able to communicate effectively.

If you are the partner in the supporting parent's role, you may have greater functioning and the ability to regulate during difficult conversations. Do your best to maintain compassion, help your partner co-regulate, and model strong communication skills if your partner approaches you harshly. If you are also stretched thin and depleted of mental and physical faculties, the self-care strategies in the next chapter can benefit you as well.

Prioritizing your relationship, working together to find ways to meet each other's needs (after your baby's needs are looked after), and interacting fondly with each other can foster greater satisfaction and connection between new parents. To help you break away from maladaptive communication patterns that leave both you and your partner feeling stuck in a negative space, here are five reminders for effective communication:

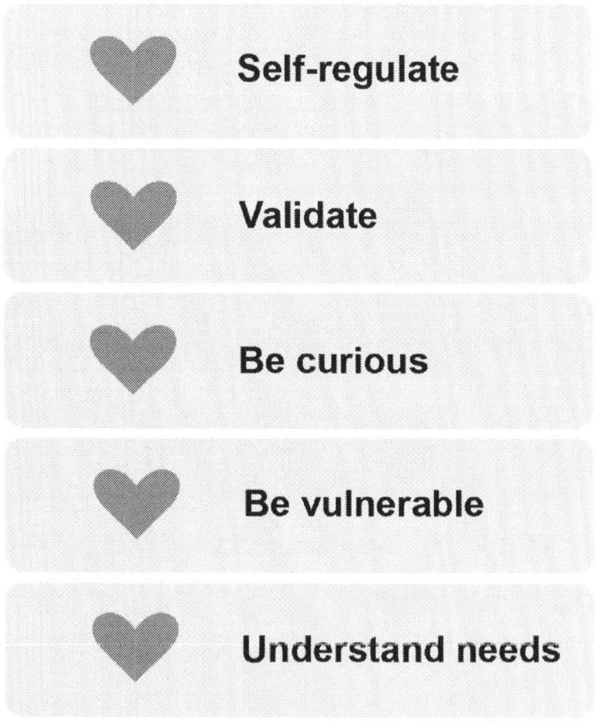
Self-regulate
Validate
Be curious
Be vulnerable
Understand needs

1. **Self-regulate:** During a heated exchange, your right (emotional) brain can overfunction as your mind and body perceive a threat and enter survival mode, destabilizing your nervous system. Therefore, you may react with a fight, flight, freeze, or fawn response to your partner. In order to remember and implement communication tools, your left (thinking) brain needs to function. Therefore, engage in emotion regulation techniques (page 91 and page 99) to help balance your nervous system, which will allow your left and right brain to reintegrate and function together.

2. **Validate:** Once you are regulated, validate your partner. You don't need to agree with what they are saying, but it will go a long way to acknowledge your partner's feelings. This will usually help them soften towards you because they will feel heard and understood. Recall that validation (page 107) recognizes your partner's feelings as being real to them, and it is not negated by your own perception of how they should or should not feel. Your perspective can be different and is also valid, but try to hold off on sharing it right out of the gate, and focus instead on acknowledging your partner's perspective. This will help to regulate them as they begin to feel seen, heard, and understood by you.

3. **Be curious:** If validation seems difficult, ask your partner questions non-defensively with a sincere desire to understand their perspective—to see things through their eyes. Avoid the urge to argue, debate, or counter their perspective by reminding yourself that this is your partner's reality, and their reality can be different than yours. Accepting that you both can experience things differently is more productive than challenging your partner's perspective. Be compassionate, be respectful, and be curious. Listen to your partner with the intention of *understanding* them instead of reacting to what they are saying.

Remember, sincere curiosity makes it possible for you to receive and absorb new information. As you process the new information, it creates opportunities for new perspectives, learning, and growth.

4. **Be vulnerable**: Share your vulnerable feelings as this can help to increase compassion, understanding, and connection between the two of you. To help you identify and communicate your vulnerable feelings, refer to the section on page 100.

5. **Understand needs**: Try to identify your partner's unmet needs when they share their concerns or feelings with you and ask how you can meet their needs better. If your partner is unable to articulate their needs, ask them what you could do differently next time to avoid the current distress in your relationship.

I wholeheartedly acknowledge how difficult it is to implement some of my suggestions. You are likely sleep deprived, low on patience, and physically and emotionally tired from looking after your baby's needs. In fact, you might be feeling exhausted at this very moment as you read these words. To a great extent, I can relate to many of your struggles as I went through them as a mother and continue to go through even as I write this book. However, as I remind myself and the couples I see in my practice, it is important to make conscious efforts after birth to maintain (or improve) relationship satisfaction with whatever energy you can muster. With everything parents do for their precious children, the greatest gift a couple can give their child is the gift of a happy, healthy, and secure relationship. Let's move forward with sensitivity in exploring the challenges of infertility and loss by reading the courageous story of a woman I am calling "Natalie."

Infertility, Loss, and Grief

We began trying to have a baby six years ago. After a few months of not being able to conceive, we went to an infertility specialist where I learned I have Polycystic Ovary Syndrome (PCOS). Because I don't ovulate every month, the doctor gave me medication to help with ovulation and increase my chances of conceiving. At this time, my husband and I were hopeful because we now knew what the issue was and the steps we needed to take to manage it. The medication was really taxing, and I had huge hormonal swings. I was sensitive and grumpy. We tried that for six months, and it didn't work. Growing up, I knew my menstrual cycle wasn't regular, but I didn't realize before what this could have meant. Unfortunately, a lot of women don't realize something is wrong until they start trying to have a baby.

We decided to do a round of in vitro fertilization (IVF) treatment a year into trying because I wanted to move things along. I went into it feeling hopeful, and my husband was supportive throughout the whole process. Unfortunately, the first IVF didn't go well at all. I felt shattered. I couldn't wrap my head around the fact that out of the 30 eggs they were able to retrieve, only one survived and was able to form an embryo.

My husband and my doctor both gave me hope and suggested we do another IVF. I agreed; however, I wanted to give my body a year to heal and address any factors that could be impacting the quality of my eggs. I managed my stress levels by reducing the number of hours I worked, continued eating healthy, started taking supplements, exercised consistently, and I even tried acupuncture. My husband also did all these things with me to show his support the only way he knew how at the time.

I went into the second round of IVF feeling hopeful again because my husband and I did everything possible to set ourselves up for success. But the treatment didn't work—again. This time, I felt worse. IVF puts your body through a lot. My hormones were all over the place, and I felt depressed and lonely. Even though I had my partner supporting and encouraging me every step of the way, it was a lonely feeling because I was going through all these hormonal changes alone. I don't think anyone understood how I was feeling. I don't think anyone can understand what a woman goes through unless they've gone through IVF too.

During this time, it helped to talk to my colleague, who was also going through an IVF treatment. I was going through my second round of IVF while she was going through her first—and she conceived. That hit me. I wondered, "We were both going through exactly the same thing, then how come her body was able to conceive and mine wasn't?"

I felt I lost the one friend who understood what I was growing through because she was now in a different phase while I still wasn't pregnant. I felt really happy for her, but I felt sad for myself...I didn't understand why my body was failing me. That's when I started feeling very sad, and my symptoms of depression became worse.

For the first time, I felt my husband's disappointment too because we had put a lot of effort into this together. He didn't need to, but he did everything with me to support me. Seeing his disappointment was hard. I felt guilty...I felt miserable...I felt like a failure. I felt like I failed myself and I failed him.

We started to disconnect from each other because I couldn't cope with what I was experiencing, and my husband didn't know how to support me. I felt unmotivated. I didn't know what to do after this. I felt lost, stressed, and pathetic. I felt I was running out of time. I put on a lot of weight and neglected my health. Looking back, it was an extremely difficult time.

In retrospect, my husband might have tried to connect with me, but I pushed him away. I became an angry person, and I closed myself off to him. He would try to make me feel better by saying things like, "It doesn't matter if we can't have kids. We have each other. We can adopt kids." But it didn't help. It only made me feel worse, and I took my anger out on him.

The anger was about my body failing me. I also felt helpless and guilty for not being able to conceive when I knew how badly my husband wanted children. And it didn't help that most of my friends started having kids around that time. When my husband would try to make me feel better by telling me to stop worrying and not feel badly about it, my anger would turn into rage.

Through the anger, disappointment, guilt, and helplessness, I finally developed the courage to prepare for a third round of IVF. However, our appointments with the fertility specialist were pushed back by over a year due to the start of the pandemic. I started stressing again because I was losing time. To make things worse, I lost my usual outlets in the pandemic which normally helped me cope with stress—the distractions, the change of scenery, going to the gym. My stress and anger eventually turned into bitterness.

I decided to put everything on hold and took time out for my mental health. I visited my family and spent a few weeks with them, leaning on them for emotional support. Though my husband is supportive in many ways, he finds it difficult to sit with my emotions and offer support in the way I need it on my low days. And to be fair, I don't always know what I need and how to ask for it.

Since visiting my family, I have started feeling a little better. I am no longer bitter, but I'm still sad. At the same time, I'm hopeful again because I have something to look forward to...we have decided to proceed with the third round of IVF!

This is the story of Natalie, a woman who bravely shared her infertility journey with me. Natalie's story is one that resonates with many women who experience infertility. As the narrative demonstrates, women who experience infertility face a wide range of emotions which significantly impact their mental health. Unfortunately, this can also result in relationship dissatisfaction.

In Canada, infertility rates are calculated to be as high as about 16 percent (Bushnik et al., 2012). After months and years of trying to conceive unsuccessfully, infertile couples can experience a strain on their relationship. Infertility not only represents a stressful experience but also a traumatic one as it can bring loss and grief. Trauma ranges from failed treatments to miscarriages, high-risk pregnancies, and the loss of a child. Such experiences impact the mental health of both partners, regardless of gender, and can result in feelings of depression, guilt, loneliness, anxiety, shame, exhaustion, helplessness, and hopelessness.

There are also couples who experience a strengthened relationship due to the closeness, safety, and comfort developed in the shared experience of infertility (Sauve, Peloquin, & Brassard, 2018). However, since I am a couple's therapist specializing in perinatal mental health, couples who experience relationship distress are the ones who contact me. Therefore, I will focus on these couples and the challenges they face due to infertility, loss, trauma, and grief.

I usually hear women express more distressing thoughts and feelings related to infertility and infertility treatments than their male counterparts. This could be explained, in part, by the differences between women and men regarding infertility. My intention is not to exclude same sex couples who want children; however, due to my lack of experience working with this population, I will discuss research on heterosexual couples.

Women's motivation to seek infertility treatments has been found to come from a desire of wanting a child whereas men's motivation for treatments is typically driven by the need to fulfill a male role, as defined socially (Davidovà & Pechovà, 2014). Therefore, women may experience infertility as an inherent failure when they are unable to fulfill their desire of a child, leading to a more significant impact on their mental health. On the other hand, perhaps men don't view infertility as an inherent failure because they are more extrinsically motivated, leading to a lower impact on their mental health.

Based on the hardships couples describe to me due to infertility, loss, and trauma, I have discerned the following five areas where couples tend to experience relationship distress:

1. **Emotional connection:** Partners can begin to disconnect if a) their experience of infertility and loss is different from one another,

b) each of them copes with the hardships differently, c) they don't feel safe being vulnerable with each other or asking for support, or d) they don't adequately provide support to each other.

2. **Communication:** Negative communication patterns can develop, in part due to the lack of emotional connection. These patterns can include anger, harshness, and avoidance strategies. Hormonal treatments can play a part in decreased emotional regulation and poor conflict management among women.

3. **Physical intimacy and sexual health:** Physical intimacy can decrease as couples begin to emotionally disconnect and engage in negative communication patterns. Sex becomes less desirable as it becomes associated with negative feelings, such as stress, disappointment, anxiety, and trauma. Women also feel responsible for tracking their ovulation cycles and initiating sex, a responsibility some women don't necessarily enjoy. Sex can feel like a task to accomplish for both partners instead of an act of love, desire, and connection. Hormonal medications can also result in decreased sexual desire among women.

4. **Adjustment:** Infertility is usually an unexpected stressor on a couple's relationship. If one or both partners are unable to manage and cope with this stress, it can lead to poor communication, poor conflict management, and relationship dissatisfaction. On the other hand, when both partners are able to develop healthy coping mechanisms and receive adequate support from one another, it can increase feelings of self-compassion, acceptance, gratitude, and closeness.

5. **Coping:** When two partners cope with infertility, loss, trauma, or grief individually, it can lead to emotional disconnection. However, when a couple is able to cope with the hardships together by

sharing the physical and emotional load, creating a plan for providing adequate support and creating a safe space for both partners' feelings and needs, it can lead to reduced stress and increased emotional connection. When both partners are able to help each other cope with an external stressor, it is referred to as dyadic coping (Bodenmann, 1995). This is a topic on which I have contributed a chapter in the book, *Couples Coping with Stress: A Cross-Cultural Perspective* (Bodenmann et al., 2016).

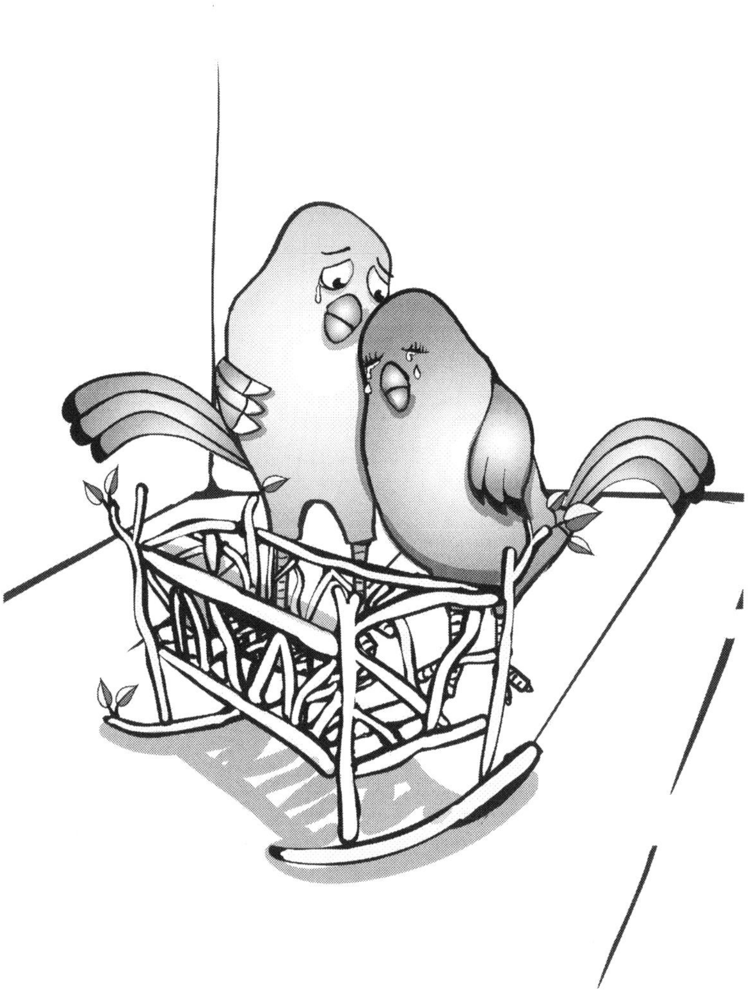

Since these are the five areas of relationship distress I usually find among couples experiencing infertility, loss, trauma, or grief, I help couples focus on improving these areas to increase their relationship strength and satisfaction. Understandably, this may be a daunting list to consider working through on your own at a time when you are already going through something difficult. For this reason, I recommend enlisting the help of a couple's therapist who specializes in infertility, trauma, and sexual health to help you strengthen the aforementioned areas in your relationship. For some of you, it may also be beneficial to consider individual therapy to help you make sense of what you are experiencing, overcome trauma, develop healthy coping skills, and learn how to ask for support while also providing support to your partner.

Finding support resources outside of your relationship can also help couples adjust and cope, reducing the pressure and strain on the relationship. Consider turning to a family member, a friend, a support group, or anyone who has faced similar struggles as you. Educating yourself on the topic using credible sources can increase your knowledge, provide you answers, help you make sense of your situation, and help you formulate a plan with your partner to manage issues related to infertility, trauma, and sexual health. I have provided a few resources in Chapter 6 to help you get started.

If you want to strengthen your relationship on your own, I recommend using the tools and guidance provided to you on attachment styles, needs, and communication in Chapter 2 and Chapter 3. I encourage you to speak to each other with compassion, vulnerability, and a desire to understand and support one another as you experience infertility and/or loss together. Avoid maladaptive behaviors such as distancing, avoiding, aggression, numbing, drinking, and substance use. Instead, turn to your partner for comfort with respect, kindness, and compassion. More than anything, work as a team to find ways to cope in healthy ways with an issue you are both facing together. Each of you may find comfort in different coping skills, and that's okay. Be understanding and supportive of one another to foster healing while maintaining closeness and connection.

You can also create a plan to help meet each other's needs and support one another in developing healthy coping strategies. For example, you may decide to take turns every week caring for any children you may have already while one of you steps away to attend therapy, a support group, meet with a friend, or engage in an activity that brings you respite. Or you may agree to engage in one of these coping strategies with your partner to provide them support, even if it isn't what helps you feel better.

Another example of coping together is creating an understanding between both of you to be accessible and responsive if one of you is feeling overwhelmed with stress, grief, or sadness. You may also decide on utilizing co-regulation strategies in moments of distress. Dyadic coping has been found to increase physical health, well-being, relationship satisfaction (Weitkamp et al., 2021), and marital quality (Bodenmann et al., 2006) and adjustment (Molgora et al., 2019). As you learn how to cope, be mindful of the long-term functionality of a coping strategy. For example, certain ways of coping, such as escaping (Rockliff et al., 2014) or avoiding (Peterson et al., 2008) have been found to be dysfunctional as they are associated with increased emotional distress and decreased marital adjustment.

To demonstrate how a couple can communicate and learn to cope together when they are feeling disconnected, I will share the story of Eric and Jessica, a married couple who has been struggling to conceive for the past four years. They have completed two rounds of IVF; the first round was unsuccessful, and the second resulted in a miscarriage. Jessica has become quiet ever since, withdrawing due to the challenging process of facing her fears. As a result, she doesn't seem interested in wanting to do things with Eric. Eric has been feeling worried, not understanding the changes in his wife's behavior.

Here is a dialogue between the spouses where Eric approaches Jessica to understand her better while remaining compassionate, respectful, and curious:

Eric:
"Jess, you want to watch a movie tonight?"

Jessica:
"Not really. I'm in the mood to read and then head to bed. I've got an early morning tomorrow."

Eric:
"I noticed you have been avoiding me lately. Whenever I ask to do something together with you, you tell me you're busy or you're not in the mood. It feels like we have been drifting apart and I'm starting to fear what this means. Can you help me understand why you don't want to do things with me anymore?"

Jessica:
"I don't feel like talking about this. I'm going to bed… I'm tired."

Eric:
"This is an example of you avoiding me again. I understand you are tired, yet, this is something very important for me to talk about with you. Can you please stay for a bit and help me understand what's going on?"

Jessica:
"Anytime we talk about our relationship, we get into an argument. It's draining and that's why I'd rather go to bed."

Eric:
"Okay, I hear your concern. I know I tend to get upset when we talk about these things. How about we talk about it, and if it starts to escalate, we agree to stop and try again later?"

Jessica:
"Okay."

Eric:
"Why don't you feel like hanging out with me anymore?"

Jessica:
"I don't know. I feel disconnected from you and it feels like I'm pretending to be normal when I'm around you. I find that exhausting."

Eric:
"I'm not sure I understand. Why do you feel the need to pretend?"

Jessica remains quiet for a few moments, visibly looking like she's holding back tears. Eric begins to feel uncomfortable and has a strong urge to say something funny to lighten the mood. He has been learning to work through his discomfort with emotions in therapy. Because of this, he is aware of what he is experiencing and instead makes a conscious decision to reach out to hold his wife's hand as he quietly moves closer to her. Jessica feels Eric's comforting presence, and leans into her husband's body as tears begin to roll down her face.

Jessica:
"Eric, I'm devastated… I have dreamt of the day I will hold a baby in my arms, and yet, there is no baby in my arms after all these years of trying!"

Eric:
"Honey, I also feel very sad that we haven't been able to have a baby but -"

Jessica:
"That's just it, Eric. It's not 'we'. It's me! I have not been able to have a baby. You're not the problem. I am. And you have no idea how that feels."

Eric:
"I don't see it that way. I have told you this before - I don't

blame you for this. This isn't your fault. I am very sad we haven't been able to have a baby but I will never blame you for this."

Jessica:

"But why don't you talk to me about these things? How come you pretend like everything's fine when it isn't?"

Eric:

"Because I don't see the point in talking and crying about something that isn't in our control."

Jessica:

"That's the problem, Eric. That is why I feel so alone and disconnected from you. I feel like I am going through this alone. I feel so much pain, so much sadness. I feel guilty. I feel angry. Somedays I feel like I want to run away from my life and never come back. And then you act normal in front of me and I have to pretend like I am normal too. And I'm tired of doing that."

Eric:

"Why don't you share these things with me?"

Jessica:

"Because whenever I have, you try to cheer me up and change the topic."

Eric:

"But if you're feeling down, shouldn't I cheer you up?"

Jessica:

"No, I don't want to be cheered up. Not in those moments."

Eric:

"Then what can I do to help you when you feel sad?"

Jessica:

"Just be with me. Listen to me, let me cry, hug me. And tell

me that you're feeling sad too. I want to know that you are also affected by this. At least I won't feel so alone anymore. I will feel like we are in this together."

Eric:
"We are in this together. You need to know that."

Jessica:
"But I don't know that. I need to hear these things from you when I am feeling low."

Eric:
"Okay, I realize now I wasn't handling the situation correctly before. I love you and I miss our time together. I will do my part to make sure I am there for you the way you need me to be. Please be patient as I will try. You know I am not very good with feelings."

Jessica:
"I know. And I appreciate your efforts to cheer me up. Deep down, I know you mean well whenever you have tried to change the topic. But it's not what helps me feel better."

Eric:
"I will try my best going forward."

Jessica and Eric quietly hug for a few moments. Each partner feels heard and understood in this exchange. Eric feels proud of himself for being able to hold space for his wife's feelings and being able to listen to her and understand her needs - something he has not been good with before. To deepen the connection he felt in this interaction, Eric asks, "*You want to watch a movie tonight?"*

Jessica feels validated, less alone, and more connected. She laughs as she responds, *"I don't want to, but I will. I miss us too!"*

As I end this section, I want to remind you grief is not a linear process that can be handled in tidy stages. It can be messy, exhausting, and complex. Grief shows up in many different ways, ranging from sadness and tears to rage and anger. Please be kind, loving, and patient with yourself and your partner as you find ways to cope and manage this time in your life. I also want to recognize those couples who come from cultures that don't have a model for grief. For these couples, it can feel shameful to express sadness. I hope you and your partner are able to create a safe and accepting space for each other to process your grief. If you are not able to, I hope you can find other relationship(s) in your life that can offer you safety and acceptance, such as with a family member, a friend, a support group, or a therapist.

This chapter covered a variety of common postpartum issues, including infertility and loss, that new parents and couples may experience. While I have provided tips and guidance on how you can learn to communicate and manage these issues, I understand the need some couples may have for additional support. For this reason, I have created workshops to expand on these topics and provide you supplemental help. You can sign up for a workshop by visiting my website: https://www.myottawatherapist.com.

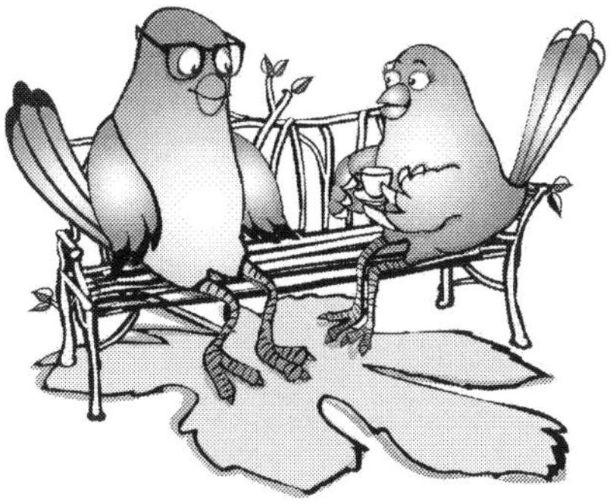

Reflections

What resonated for you in this chapter?

What are the key points you want to remember?

What might be worth discussing with your partner?

What tool or strategy do you want to put into practice?

Chapter 5: *Self-Care*

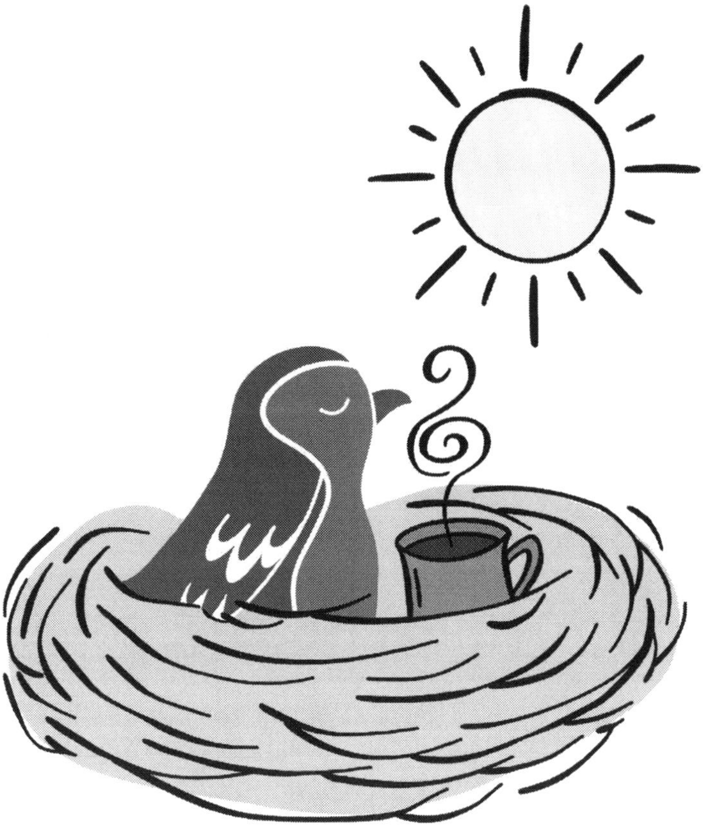

What Is Self-Care?

If you scroll through social media, self-care seems to mean bubble baths, massages, and wine time. While these activities are enjoyable for some people, self-care is much deeper and bigger than that from a mental health perspective. When I talk about self-care with clients, I'm referring to an action, or a set of actions, that needs to be taken by the client to protect their mental and emotional health. For some, self-care can mean taking a nap to rejuvenate their mind, body, and spirit. For others, it also means:

- Embracing imperfection
- Replacing self-criticisms with self-compassion
- Setting healthy boundaries
- Taking a break
- Decluttering your space
- Ending toxic cycles
- Seeking therapy to support your mental health
- Practicing good sleep and eating habits
- Going out for walks or exercising
- Saying "no"
- Taking out time to do something you enjoy outside of parenting
- Choosing who to spend time with
- Connecting with a higher power, spirituality, or meditation
- Attuning to your emotional needs and fulfilling them
- Aligning with your values to bring you peace
- Prioritizing your physical and mental health

With couples who are in the postpartum period, I often find conversations of self-care stemming from discussions of lacking good boundaries, unmet expectations, sensory overload, and feelings of self-doubt and guilt. Therefore, these are the topics I will expand upon in this chapter in the context of self-care.

Establishing Boundaries

Healthy boundaries are one of the main components of self-care. It can also be a challenging topic for many couples. Without boundaries, feelings of frustration, anger, resentment, and exhaustion can take place, eventually leading to burnout. Boundaries help us maintain a sense of self and provide balance in work, life, and relationships. Before we can establish healthy boundaries, we first must understand what they are and what their purpose is.

Boundaries are the rules of a relationship, set by the people involved. This includes the relationship you have with yourself, which I will explain later in this section. These rules are created based on what each person is comfortable or not comfortable with. The level of comfort for each person depends on their set of values, principles, attachment style, and belief systems. Boundaries range from rigid to no boundary, with a healthy boundary falling somewhere in between the two. When you communicate and consistently maintain your boundaries, it teaches others what your limits are and how to interact with you. When you don't communicate or consistently maintain your boundaries, it either teaches others that you don't have limits, or it confuses them when your limits are inconsistent. Boundaries also help you maintain your identity and autonomy. In other words, your sense of self remains intact in a relationship with healthy boundaries.

A person's sense of self is usually based on their self-worth and self-esteem. Thus, people who have a fragile sense of self are often uncertain about their boundaries or how to express and maintain boundaries. Unfortunately, the uncertainty or inability to uphold boundaries reaffirms low self-worth and low self-esteem.

When explaining boundaries to my clients, I liken them to the entrance of a house. Imagine the front door of your house is shut tightly at all times regardless of who or what approaches it; this doesn't allow anyone or anything to enter your house at any point. Your house inside remains untouched, unchanged, and uninfluenced. You have complete control. Now imagine your front door is open wide; this allows anyone and anything to enter your home, creating the opportunity for your house to be affected, changed, or influenced in any manner whether by a person, rain, wind, or a stray cat. You have no control.

Finally, imagine you have a screen door which is closed, but the front door behind it remains open; this allows the elements you would like to open your home to, such as fresh air, scenery, and an opportunity to say "hello" to neighbors walking by. However, it keeps out intruders, stray animals, and anyone or anything else that makes you feel uncomfortable entering inside your house. Having a screen door also gives you flexibility in deciding whether or not you are comfortable with letting someone or something in based on changing circumstances. Hence, having a healthy boundary is like having a screen door.

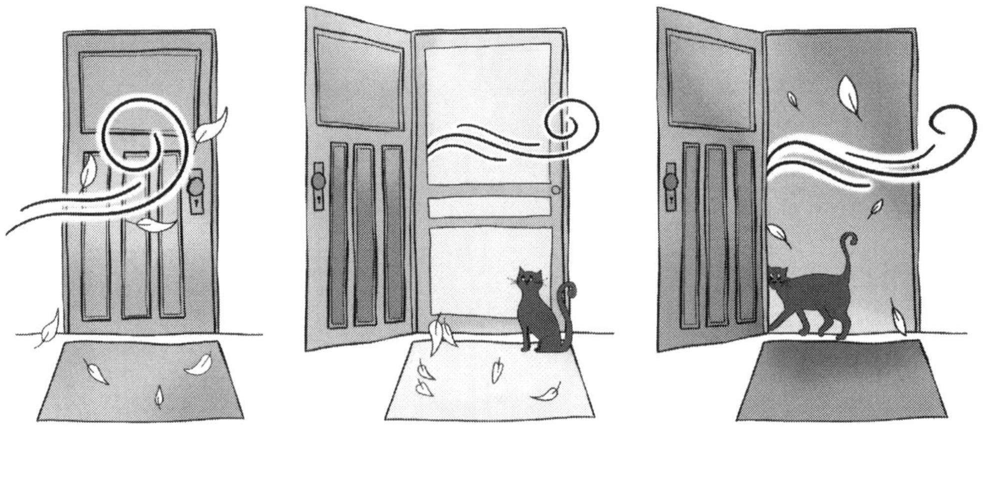

Before I talk about different types of boundaries, I want to highlight that you are responsible for setting and maintaining your own boundaries. In other words, as an adult, a boundary is *your* responsibility to ensure *your* physical and mental health. No adult has the authority to decide what another adult's boundaries should be because each person's level of comfort is personal and unique to them. Therefore, every adult who is of sound mind and health is responsible for identifying, communicating, and maintaining their own boundaries. Furthermore, boundaries are not meant to control other people's behaviors or create distances in relationships. Rather, they are meant to create understanding, trust, and safety between two people, which can also lead to more closeness and connection within a relationship.

Boundaries with Yourself

When the discussion arises on how to set boundaries with others, I remind my clients that they must also learn to set boundaries with themselves. To expect other people to understand and respect your comfort levels, you must also expect that of yourself in order to maintain good physical and mental health.

Here are examples of important self-boundaries new parents can consider during pregnancy, and especially during the postpartum months:

1. Setting limits with yourself. This includes managing time spent on your phone or on social media, how many projects or assignments you take on at work, or the number of episodes you watch before going to sleep.
2. Prioritizing your sleep and your nutrition. For example, going to sleep at a regular time every night and eating nutritious meals at regular intervals during the day.
3. Allowing yourself breaks by leaning on your partner, a family member, a friend, or a babysitter for help.
4. Learning to manage your time well to avoid stressful situations.
5. Ending toxic patterns of thoughts and feelings, such as guilt, anger, rage, self-criticisms, excessive worry, and more.
6. Ensuring good physical hygiene. For some, that may include changing into fresh clothes every morning before starting the day.

7. Carving out time to connect with meaningful adult relationships. This can include going out for a walk with a friend or family member once a week or giving them a call if going out with your baby seems challenging.
8. Meeting with a psychotherapist routinely to support you in regaining and maintaining good mental health.
9. Overcoming an addiction with the help of a professional.
10. Limiting self-deprecating thoughts and increasing self-compassion, especially if you are finding it difficult to engage in self-care.

Boundaries with yourself sound like this:

- *"I will choose to go to sleep at 10 p.m. tonight and every night from now on. Anything that is left to be done, I will do it tomorrow."*
- *"I will ask for help when I start to feel overwhelmed."*
- *"I will politely decline anything that requires more time and energy from me."*
- *"I will set my alarm to wake up 30 minutes before the baby every morning so I can have a few moments to myself to start the day with positivity and gratitude."*
- *"I will stop after one drink tonight."*
- *"I will prioritize eating breakfast every morning."*
- *"I will walk away from negative interactions before I lose control of my emotions. I will practice self-regulation and return to the conversation once I am able to engage more effectively."*

Boundaries with Your Partner

A tenet of a healthy relationship is two people's ability to set and maintain healthy boundaries with compassion. Couples who have a stable and secure foundation in their relationship usually have a set of rules, or healthy boundaries, they both understand and respect. Ideally, these rules are clearly defined and communicated during the early stages of the relationship, reducing opportunity for misunderstandings, hurt feelings, or a loss of trust and safety in the relationship. Remember, a boundary is not an ultimatum or a threat. Rather, it is you discussing and sharing what your personal boundaries are so that those around you understand.

Communicating your boundaries and reevaluating them as the relationship evolves can result in deepened understanding between two partners, creating a sense of certainty and predictability. Boundaries also establish a mutual understanding where both partners are aware of the limits they cannot cross with each other. This helps to maintain stability, safety, and security in the relationship. Finally, as healthy boundaries cultivate mutual understanding and respect between two partners, they also increase a couple's emotional intimacy with each other. Emotional intimacy is a couple's deep sense of knowing each other beyond what others know of them, respecting each other, feeling safe and protected with one another, and lovingly accepting differences.

While healthy boundaries should exist in every relationship, including in a marriage, it is a balancing act between developing closeness and maintaining autonomy. When one or both partners begin to lose their sense of identity and autonomy in a relationship, it can result in "enmeshment"—a term coined by family therapist Salvadore Minuchin (1974). Enmeshment is the idea that two people are entangled with each other to a point where you can no longer determine where one person's thoughts, feelings, and opinions end, and the other person's begin. On the other hand, too much distance in a relationship can result in disconnection and separate lives.

In a couple's relationship, having a boundary is simply letting your partner know what you are comfortable with and what you are not comfortable with. It is respectfully making your partner aware of your limits, what makes you feel safe, and what keeps you feeling physically and mentally healthy. At the same time, it is being open to understanding and respecting your partner's needs and boundaries as well.

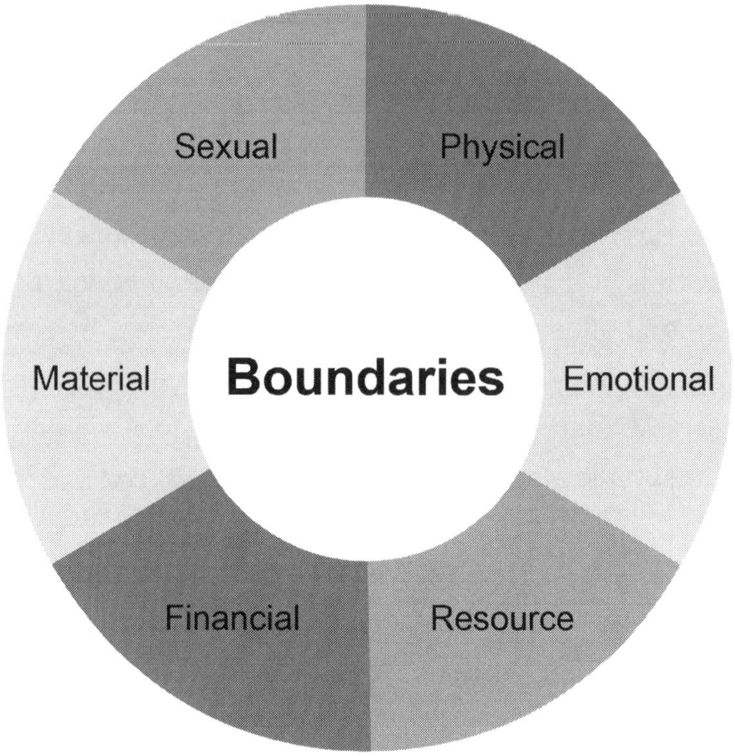
Sexual
Physical
Material
Boundaries
Emotional
Financial
Resource

The following are six different types of boundaries most relevant in a couple's relationship, and examples of how you can communicate them lovingly but firmly:

1. **Physical:** This includes your personal space and the type of touch you are okay or not okay with.

    - *"I know you mean well when you hug me if I am frustrated. However, I do not like to be touched when I am angry."*
    - *"Please knock before you come in."*
    - *"I prefer a shoulder rub versus a foot rub because my feet are ticklish."*
    - *"I love it when you are affectionate with me. However, I feel uncomfortable in public. I prefer we show affection to each other in the privacy of our home."*

2. **Emotional:** This includes the amount of emotional energy you have in your reserves to give to someone else, how much emotional energy you are able to receive from someone else before feeling drained, being treated with respect, and knowing your limits on what and how much to share.

    - *"Please don't yell at me. I don't like the way it makes me feel."*
    - *"I need to walk away for a few minutes and cool off before we can talk about this."*
    - *"It sounds like you had a tough day at work. I want to be here for you, but right now, I am not in the right frame of mind. Can we talk later tonight?"*
    - *"I love your humor and how you make me laugh, but I don't find it funny when you poke fun at me as a mother. It is a sensitive topic for me. I want to be taken more seriously while I'm figuring out how to be a good parent."*
    - *"I will find it easier to listen to you once I am able to finish what I am trying to share with you. Please hear me out without interrupting."*

3. **Resources:** This includes your time, physical energy, knowledge, and skills.

    - *"I will not be able to help you this week, I have a lot on my plate. Can we set up a time for next week?"*
    - *"No, I am sorry. I cannot do that."*
    - *"I love this idea; however, the timing won't work. When the baby is napping, it is the only time I have to myself. I hope you can understand how necessary this time is for me."*
    - *"I need to sleep early on weeknights. I'll watch shows with you on the weekends."*

4. **Financial:** This includes your personal finances, your level of comfort with sharing finances, and making financial decisions.

    - *"I am not okay with our joint account being used for spending on things that we have not agreed upon. Let's agree to communicate with each other before making a big purchase."*
    - *"I will need transparency regarding how much debt you have before we get married."*
    - *"Can we sit down together sometime this week to reevaluate how to split the bills and expenses between us? I am unable to keep up with my share of the responsibility with the maternity benefits I receive."*

5. **Material:** This includes the use of your personal possessions.

    - *"Please don't look through my phone. If you have any concerns, you can ask me directly. I would like my privacy to be respected the same way I respect yours."*
    - *"I hope you can understand how frustrating it is when I can't find something in its usual place. Going forward, please return things where you found them."*

6. **Sexual:** This includes your comfort and your consent when it comes to different types of touch and acts of intimacy.

    - *"Our sex life is important to me, and I want to help you understand what feels best for me and what I don't like."*
    - *"I don't like how that feels; this feels better to me instead."*
    - *"It's been a rough day. I am not in the mood tonight."*
    - *"Stop."*
    - *"No."*

- *"It turns me off when you call me that name. I know you are being playful, but I don't like it."*

Not all of these boundaries have to be part of your relationship. Boundaries are determined by what is important to you, what helps you feel comfortable with another person, and what you need in order to establish trust and safety. It can be hard to figure out what your boundaries are, especially if you grew up without healthy boundaries modeled to you by caregivers. It can also be difficult to recognize what your boundaries are if they have been disregarded or violated in the past.

How to Determine Your Boundaries

You can determine your boundaries by becoming aware of your physiological responses, emotions, thoughts, and behaviors in certain situations or around particular people. You can increase self-awareness by reflecting back on experiences you have had throughout your life and focusing on the ones that stand out to you as being uncomfortable. If this seems difficult, start by focusing on uncomfortable situations in the past few months. Out of these experiences, what are some common patterns you can ascertain? Upon reflection, you might recognize there is a pattern in your life similar to one or more of the following examples:

- Feelings of discomfort when someone enters your physical space without your permission
- Increased feelings of anxiety when you are around a particular person at work
- Feeling overwhelmed in certain types of situations
- A pounding in your ears and blood rushing to your face each time someone from your family questions your style of parenting
- Feeling anxious around one of your parents
- Avoiding a particular person, situation, or topic repeatedly in your life

- Not feeling safe to speak your mind in a relationship
- Feeling angry when you are taken advantage of
- Feeling resentment towards someone after agreeing to help them
- Dodging calls from a friend or feeling anxious when they text you
- Feeling nervous and walking on eggshells with your partner
- Feeling as if you are choking back tears

Once you are able to determine what your boundaries are, begin establishing them. I recommend starting with a relationship that feels safe —or less risky. For example, you may decide it is safer to practice communicating a boundary with a co-worker before doing so with your manager. Or you may want to practice setting one with a friend before setting one with your partner. Remember, upholding a boundary with a person is not about controlling their behavior. It is *your* boundary, meaning it is there to identify your limits to others, recognize when a limit is being crossed, and decide on what *you* would like to do about it to maintain comfort and safety.

If you find yourself still uncertain about your boundaries, you can observe the boundaries maintained by others around you by paying attention to how people react or respond to particular topics, situations, or people. You can even ask close friends or family members about what boundaries they uphold in their life. This can give you ideas about what boundaries you might like to establish in your life to maintain good physical and mental health. Finally, working with a therapist can help you determine your boundaries and teach you how to communicate them.

How to Communicate Boundaries

The best way to communicate a boundary is clearly, respectfully, and consistently. It can be tricky to set boundaries in close relationships, especially if you have not done it before. Therefore, I also encourage my clients to be patient and gentle while remaining firm when establishing their boundaries in close relationships.

As explained extensively in Chapter 3, using blaming language can result in your partner or any other person responding in a reactive manner to you. Therefore, I suggest keeping the focus on yourself instead of pointing fingers when articulating the following to establish your boundary:

1. How you feel about an issue
2. Why you feel this way
3. What you prefer happens instead the next time
4. What you will do to maintain your boundary if it is disregarded

To demonstrate, here is an example of how you can communicate a boundary to your partner, without pointing fingers:

"I feel worried when we start yelling in front of the kids. It is important for me to ensure our kids do not witness us becoming aggressive towards each other. Therefore, the next time this happens, I will respectfully remind us both to lower our voices. If we are struggling to de-escalate, I will let you know I'm stepping away from the conversation and will wait to continue it with you after the kids are in bed and we both have cooler heads."

Here is another example:

"I feel angry when the TV is turned on in our room when I am trying to sleep at night. The baby keeps me up most of the night, and I need to sleep early, otherwise I wake up tired and cranky the next day. You have noticed it too—you pointed this out to me yesterday when I was impatient and snappy with you. I was thinking about a plan that might work for us both. How about we watch an episode together in bed and then turn off the TV by 10 p.m.? If you forget or decide to watch another episode, I will

remind you how important it is for me to sleep early in order to be more patient with you and our baby the next day. What do you think? Does this sound like a reasonable plan to you?"

While I recommend establishing boundaries clearly, respectfully, and consistently, I will also stress the importance of open-ended and compassionate discussions in your close relationships. Your partner may not understand you at first and may have some questions for you. They may even feel confused or hurt with your boundary, which is not uncommon. They may test or push back on your stated boundary - again, this is not unusual at the start. To be open and willing to discuss a boundary does not mean you need to compromise it. Instead, what it means is you understand your partner is human and may require patience and time to process and respect the new boundary.

The key to helping your partner or another person learn to regard your boundaries is by 1) explaining to them ahead of time what you will do to maintain your boundary if it's being pushed or ignored, and 2) following through with it. By honoring your plan to uphold your boundary, you are demonstrating how important the boundary is to you and how serious you are about protecting your physical and mental health.

HOW TO SET A BOUNDARY

- ☑ Identify your feeling(s) about an issue.
- ☑ Explain the concern or discomfort you have with the issue.
- ☑ Identify boundary: Share what you prefer happens instead next time.
- ☑ Set a consequence: Highlight the importance of the boundary.
- ☑ Keep it simple: Avoid the need to over explain.

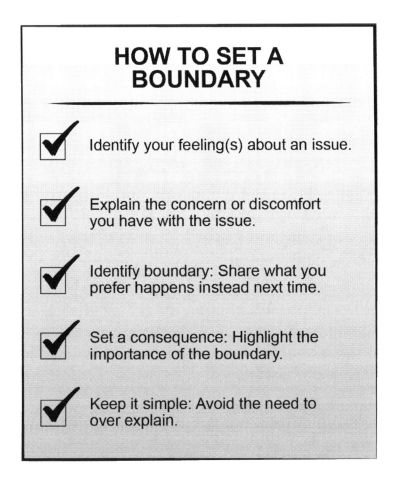

Unhealthy versus Healthy Boundaries

This is a good time to explain the difference between unhealthy and healthy boundaries. If you tend to have rigid boundaries, it means you set and maintain unwavering, inflexible, and possibly unreasonable boundaries which remain the same no matter what the context of a situation is, or who the person is. It leaves no room for perspective, understanding, compassion, or flexibility. Unfortunately, rigid boundaries can result in poor mental health as well as distance and disconnection in relationships. Thus, rigid boundaries are unhealthy.

If you tend to have loose boundaries, it means there is no consistency in how you establish your boundaries, who you establish them with, and what methods you use to maintain them—if at all. This results in people receiving mixed messages from you and not knowing how or which boundaries to respect. Therefore, this negatively impacts your mental health because you don't consistently feel comfortable or safe in relationships. For these reasons, loose boundaries are also unhealthy.

If you tend to have flexible boundaries, it means there is a clear pattern and consistency with which you establish and maintain them. You communicate your boundaries firmly, but you allow room to adjust your expectations around the boundary once you determine that adjusting may in fact be more beneficial than harmful to your mental health. This is what differentiates flexible boundaries from rigid ones, and what makes them healthier. This is not to say that you compromise your safety or comfort. Instead, it is being open to assessing your level of safety and comfort in specific circumstances or in certain relationships and making a decision to maintain or adjust your boundary accordingly.

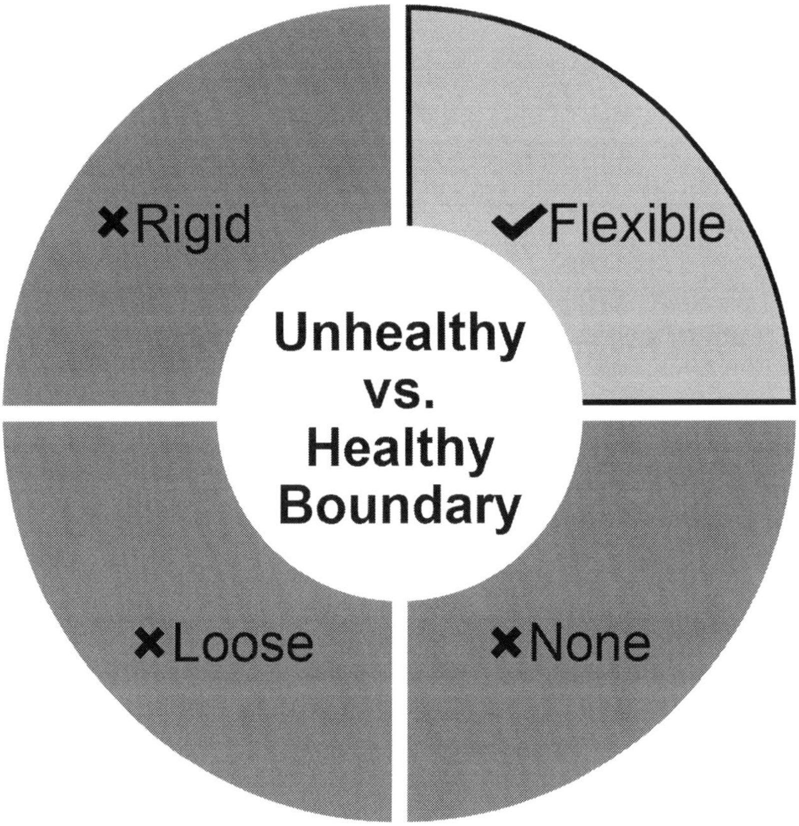
✖Rigid
✔Flexible
Unhealthy
vs.
Healthy
Boundary
✖Loose
✖None

To give an obvious example, consider you have a boundary around personal space. However, if you are in a crowded area or a cramped space, such as a concert or public transport, you will probably let go of the expectation that no one can enter your personal space. In these scenarios, it will be crucial for you to understand the context and also understand the difference between someone *violating* your personal space versus someone simply being *in* your personal space because there isn't enough space to begin with. In this case, you might find it beneficial to reevaluate your safety and adjust your expectations around your boundary if someone stands close to you without ill intent.

I will share a personal example to explain flexible boundaries further: I have established a boundary firmly around bedtime for my children; they know when it is time to eat their dinner, brush their teeth, read a story, and sleep. This is a boundary I set very early in motherhood when my eldest was a baby. I set this boundary for my own sanity, and it required clear and repeated communication with my husband so he understood its importance.

I explained to my husband that it was important to create a boundary to ensure our baby slept earlier in the evenings and also got to spend quiet time with one of us alone about an hour before it was time for him to sleep. I created this boundary because my son used to cry inconsolably for hours almost every night for the first two months of his life. It was draining and painful to watch. I felt helpless every evening, desperately trying anything to soothe him and stop the crying. I also felt very anxious as a new mother in front of my in-laws who witnessed his crying in the early days during their frequent visits.

Once I was able to (somewhat) have my wits about me as a new mother, I began doing research to understand why my newborn was crying in the evenings and what I could do to help him. I soon learned about the infamous "witching hour," which refers to the hour every evening where many babies cry inconsolably due to overstimulation or being over tired. Thus, the boundary around my son's bedtime became very important, not only for my mental health, but also for my baby's physical and mental health.

At first, I don't think my husband fully appreciated how this boundary was necessary to help my son and to help me cope with my anxiety and stress in the evenings. I don't think our family members fully understood either. But every day, without fail, I upheld this boundary by taking my son upstairs to our bedroom earlier than usual, giving him milk, reading a story, and cuddling him in our quiet room with dim lights. My husband often joined me to help, which I appreciated. I continued to follow these steps, with love and compassion, even when family members wanted to hold my son and play with him longer. I politely reminded any family member who was present why this was necessary as I would respectfully proceed to carry him upstairs at the same time every evening.

Eventually, as I consistently modeled this boundary, my son no longer cried in the evenings. As a result, it reduced my anxiety and stress levels. My husband noticed the positive changes and started to uphold the boundary himself, without needing reminders. Family members also began to understand and respect the boundary. Establishing it was one of the best decisions I have made as a mother, but it was not an overnight success. It was a process that required patience, consistency, and ongoing communication with my husband and in-laws.

As I settled into my role as a new mother, this boundary became an integral part of my self-care. The key word is "self-care"—something mothers don't always give themselves permission to practice. Raising two active toddlers in a pandemic with frequent lockdowns and an abundance of time spent together at home, suffice it to say, the only thing that got me through each day was knowing that both my children would be in bed by a certain time every evening. This created structure and routine during a monotonous time. Best of all, it created predictability in our family life, allowing both my husband and I to have much-needed quiet time alone or together as a couple.

I continue to uphold this boundary to this day, because without it, I know I will be at my wits' end at the close of each day. However, this boundary has room for flexibility because I continue to adjust it as my children grow older. For example, now that my children are older, my husband and I spend a lot of time outdoors every summer. This means we don't always eat dinner at home, nor do we always have time for a story before they sleep. As long as my children are in bed around the same time every night, how we go about their bedtime routine in the summers is flexible.

Another way this boundary is flexible is it takes into account our social plans on weekends. My husband and I usually make a plan with friends every weekend, and our children sleep later than usual if they are with us. My children also know this is one of the few conditions under which they can sleep late. This is an example of how the boundary is flexible, yet there is consistency in when, how, and with whom it is maintained. Clarity, consistency, and flexibility establishes predictability, safety, and security for my children.

A final example of how this is a firm but flexible boundary is how I adjust my expectations when we are traveling. We are outside of our usual environment when we are on a trip, and I recognize that attempting to implement a strict routine will cause me and my husband more stress than help. It will also distress my children as they will naturally struggle to follow a routine in a place that is new and exciting. In fact, upholding the usual bedtime boundary while traveling would be the direct opposite of my self-care because it would cause me daily stress trying to maintain it. Therefore, to manage our expectations of this boundary while traveling to new places, my husband and I have come to an agreement that we will do our best to ensure our children get adequate rest and sleep without watching the clock or stressing about timing. Upon return, we agree to give ourselves and our children some grace as we settle in at home and reestablish the boundary.

As you are learning, healthy boundaries are those that are firm but make room for flexibility. However, there are times in a relationship where boundaries may need to be negotiated between two people. To learn how to negotiate boundaries, let's take a look at the next section.

Negotiating Boundaries

The more intimate a relationship is, such as the one shared by a couple, the more there can be a need for respectfully negotiating boundaries so both partners can experience a balanced and comfortable relationship. A need for negotiation can arise when one partner's boundary impacts the other partner negatively. To explain this further, I will share the example of Amy and Kunle, a married couple with a 13-month-old toddler:

Amy is home all day looking after her son, Jackson. She feels grateful for being able to stay home and raise her son without any competing priorities; however, she also feels lonely. With the couple moving to a new city soon after Jackson's birth, Amy didn't have a chance to make any friends. She also doesn't have any family close by, leaving her feeling isolated and alone.

Little Jackson doesn't know how to crawl yet and likes to spend time in his mama's arms. Between carrying her son around the house all day and keeping him fed, rested, and entertained, Amy desperately looks forward to the moment she hears her husband's car pulling into the driveway every evening. She knows that as soon as Kunle's home, she can hand off Jackson to him and catch a much-needed break from baby duties. She also can't wait to talk to Kunle about her day and ask him questions about his day at work. This helps her cope with her feeling of loneliness and allows her to feel connected to her husband.

On the other hand, Kunle struggles to meet Amy's needs for connection and support with Jackson because he feels drained after a long day at work. He looks forward to coming home and having some time to himself —in silence. However, he is aware that his wife expects him to engage with her, empathize with her, and even bounce ideas together to help her manage her day better with their son. Kunle tries his best to engage with his wife but continues to feel more stressed and exhausted every evening. Lately, he has been irritable with Amy anytime she talks to him, which leaves him feeling guilty.

Kunle feels guilty for being irritable because he is the reason they relocated. He believes he should be there for Amy in whatever way she needs because she left her family and friends behind to support his career. However, since meeting with his therapist to learn how to manage his stress better, Kunle realizes how his attempts to meet Amy's needs every evening at the expense of his mental health has been causing friction between the couple and adversely impacting their relationship. With the help of his therapist, he is learning the importance of establishing a boundary while also considering Amy's needs.

The following is a dialogue between the couple which showcases how Kunle established a boundary but was also open to negotiating it in order to meet his wife's needs as well:

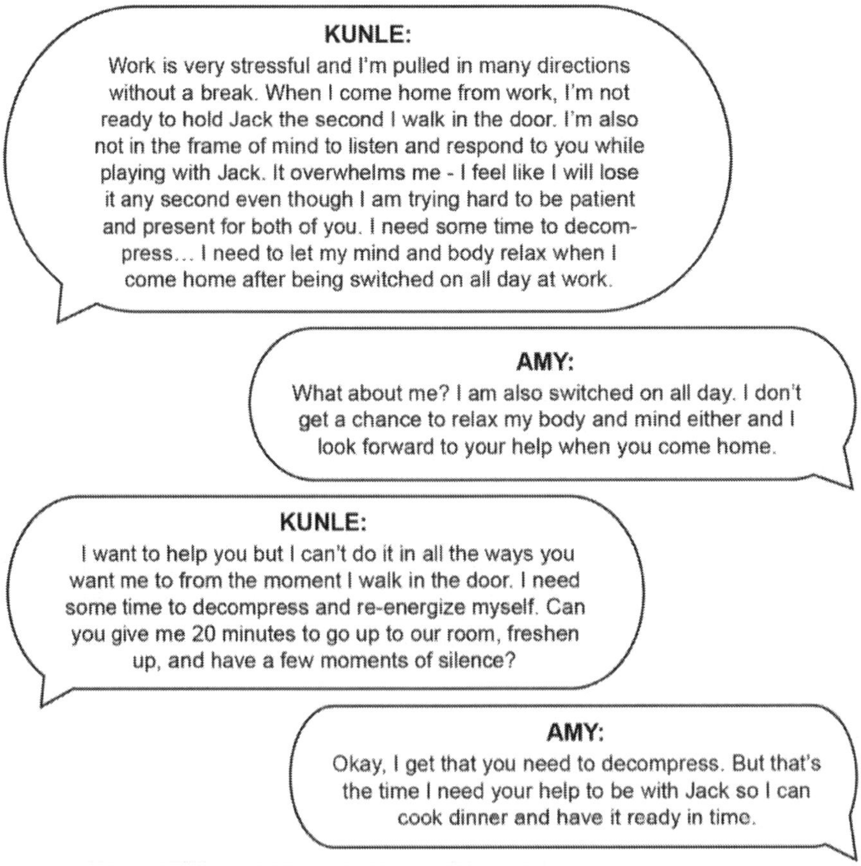
KUNLE:
Work is very stressful and I'm pulled in many directions without a break. When I come home from work, I'm not ready to hold Jack the second I walk in the door. I'm also not in the frame of mind to listen and respond to you while playing with Jack. It overwhelms me - I feel like I will lose it any second even though I am trying hard to be patient and present for both of you. I need some time to decompress… I need to let my mind and body relax when I come home after being switched on all day at work.
AMY:
What about me? I am also switched on all day. I don't get a chance to relax my body and mind either and I look forward to your help when you come home.
KUNLE:
I want to help you but I can't do it in all the ways you want me to from the moment I walk in the door. I need some time to decompress and re-energize myself. Can you give me 20 minutes to go up to our room, freshen up, and have a few moments of silence?
AMY:
Okay, I get that you need to decompress. But that's the time I need your help to be with Jack so I can cook dinner and have it ready in time.

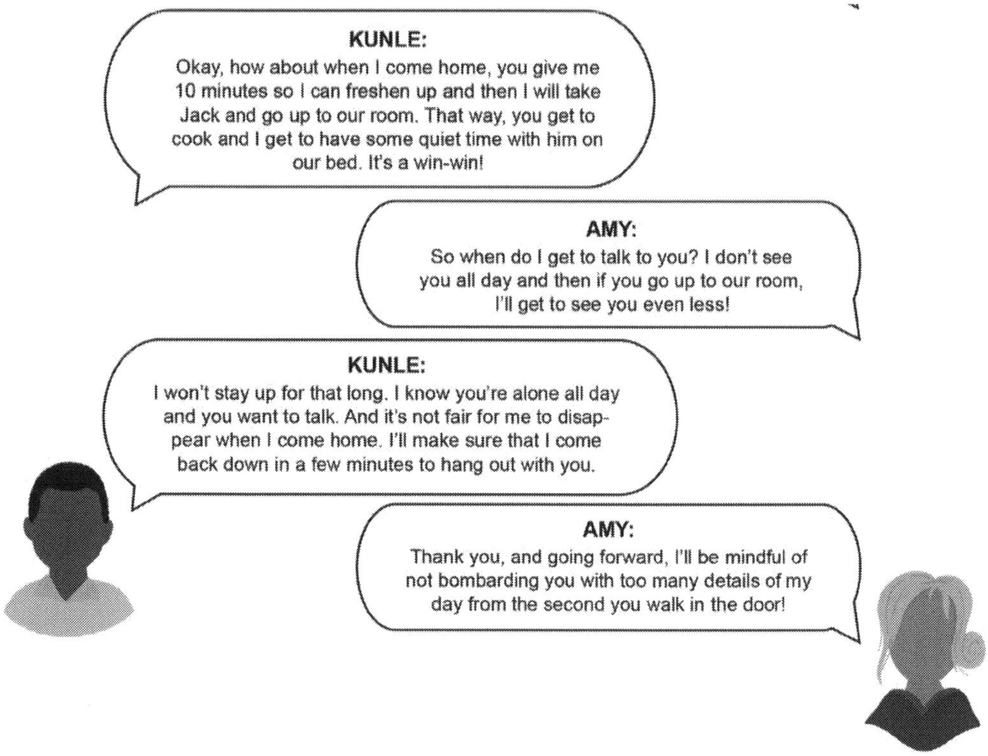
KUNLE:
Okay, how about when I come home, you give me 10 minutes so I can freshen up and then I will take Jack and go up to our room. That way, you get to cook and I get to have some quiet time with him on our bed. It's a win-win!
AMY:
So when do I get to talk to you? I don't see you all day and then if you go up to our room, I'll get to see you even less!
KUNLE:
I won't stay up for that long. I know you're alone all day and you want to talk. And it's not fair for me to disappear when I come home. I'll make sure that I come back down in a few minutes to hang out with you.
AMY:
Thank you, and going forward, I'll be mindful of not bombarding you with too many details of my day from the second you walk in the door!

Like Kunle and Amy, if you think you and your partner may benefit from negotiating boundaries to ensure you are both feeling comfortable and content around each other, here are a few questions which might be helpful to reflect upon:

- What boundaries do you need to establish to maintain good mental health in your relationship with each other?
- Are there any boundaries which are harming your shared closeness and connection?
- What will help maintain mutual closeness and connection while still honoring individual boundaries?
- How can you negotiate your boundaries so both of you enjoy good mental health, closeness, and connection?

- How much flexibility can your boundary, or boundaries, tolerate while still maintaining adequate comfort for you?

When you are negotiating boundaries, don't forget you are a team. Both of you will benefit from working together and finding ways to make the relationship mutually satisfying, safe, and comfortable. If one of you upholds your boundaries rigidly without an open and fair conversation, it will convey a disregard of your partner's feelings and needs. This may cause feelings of resentment, sadness, loneliness, and/or anger in your partner which can lead to distance and disconnection in your relationship. On the other hand, if one of you feels like you have to ignore your boundaries to please your partner, manage their feelings, or satisfy their needs, it will also lead to unpleasant emotions which can create ruptures in your relationship. Therefore, to achieve the right balance, it requires compassion, teamwork, and positive intentions.

For more guidance on negotiating boundaries, continue to read the following section where I share five steps I use to guide the conversation between couples in therapy who are attempting to negotiate a boundary.

Boundaries in Different Cultures

Each culture has its own way of understanding and establishing boundaries. Being born in a South Asian culture and growing up in North America, I have struggled, and continue to struggle, managing the tension between my belief as a therapist in the importance of setting healthy boundaries, and the perception around boundaries held by South Asians at large. The clash between my belief and my culture's perception about boundaries has been challenging and confusing for me to experience. Hence, I relate wholeheartedly to clients who struggle with the concept of establishing boundaries within their culture.

I am fortunate to have a diverse clientele and recognize the discomfort and difficulty one may experience when communicating their boundaries to others, and even oneself, due to pre-established cultural norms. To understand what I mean, consider the patriarchal cultures where hierarchy in family structure and gender role ascriptions are of utmost importance. In these cultures, there are pre-existing boundaries that are often one-directional and rigidly upheld as a cultural norm. For example, parents may have rigid boundaries around what children can or cannot say to their parents or speak to them about. However, within the same culture, it would be considered acceptable for the parents to speak to their children as they please. This applies similarly to spousal relationships, where it may be considered acceptable for a husband to have expectations of his wife and to implement consequences if his expectations are not met, but the same might not apply the other way around.

Another example is that of collectivist cultures, where group harmony and group needs are more important than individual happiness and individual needs. Within a collectivist culture, a struggling wife or a mother may consider it to be out of the question for her to establish boundaries with her husband, family, or her in-laws to protect her mental health. In this case, she would be more focused on maintaining peace and avoiding conflict instead of doing what might improve her mental health. The same would apply to a struggling husband or a father who might suppress his own feelings and needs to maintain peace in his family.

Another example is of those cultures where gender role ascriptions are strongly maintained, and rigid boundaries can exist to protect these gender roles; to go outside of the boundary would be considered a deviation from societal expectations and norms. To explain, it may be looked down upon for a man to be involved in childcare duties such as changing a diaper or feeding their baby. It may be equally frowned upon for a woman to be involved in financial matters of the household. Thus, rigid boundaries may exist within a family to maintain the traditional gender roles.

If you find yourself struggling with the idea of setting a boundary, whether with yourself, your spouse, or a family member, keep in mind that belonging to a culture does not automatically mean you must follow every norm of that culture. While following cultural norms can help you maintain your identity and provide you with a sense of belonging, it is also commonplace for people within a culture to have variations in their values and practices. In fact, within the same culture, every family has its own unique culture.

Think about it: When two people are married, they often realize they have different ways of doing some things even though they share the same racial and religious background. This is because they come from two different families who had variations in values, practices, traditions, gender role expectations, and boundaries. At some point, these two individuals will benefit from learning how to adjust, compromise, and adapt as they create their own culture as husband and wife.

As you and your partner work together to define your own culture, consider the different cultural norms you both practice. Evaluate which norms serve both of you well, help you grow as a couple, and develop a strong connection between you. Also evaluate the ones that keep you stuck in patterns that do more harm than good to your relationship and your mental health.

What is beneficial and what is harmful is unique in every relationship. For example, a couple might benefit from maintaining traditional gender roles where the husband is the breadwinner and the wife is the homemaker, whereas another couple might suffer in trying to maintain traditional gender roles. A couple might benefit from the involvement of family members, and another couple might experience harmful effects to their mental health. A couple might benefit from parenting their children the same way they were parented, and another might consider it harmful to repeat generational patterns of parenting.

Once you are able to recognize cultural practices and norms that are more harmful than beneficial to your relationship and to your mental health, identify boundaries you would like to establish in order to cultivate the culture you want to create in your new family as a couple. This includes boundaries between you and your partner and boundaries between your relationship and those people who are outside of your relationship. As I continue to elaborate on the topic of boundaries, I would like to remind you of the importance of practicing flexible (healthy) boundaries, instead of rigid or loose (unhealthy) boundaries. To review the difference, you can read the section again on page 214.

Some of you may be wondering, *This all sounds nice, but what happens when my partner and I have different ideas about which practices, traditions, and norms we want to keep? What happens when we disagree on what boundaries are important to each of us? What happens when one partner's boundary creates tension or harmful effects in the relationship?*

Naturally, there will be some differences between you and your partner. You are two different people, coming from two different sets of families and life experiences, with two different ways of thinking, perceiving, and feeling. As you have learned, *how* you communicate will matter just as much as what you are communicating about. Healthy relationships are built on a foundation of respect, compassion, and compromise. I recommend keeping these values at the forefront of your mind as you negotiate boundary setting with each other.

When I help couples respectfully negotiate boundaries, I guide their discussion through a series of steps. I suggest the same steps to help you guide your conversation:

1. **Understand why your partner has a boundary.** Boundaries are there to protect one's mental health. Therefore, understand how the boundary serves to protect your partner's mental health. If relevant, ask questions to understand the boundary in context of their cultural and religious background, even if you share the same background. Remember that when asking questions, you are seeking to learn and understand, not debate or negate. As I pointed out earlier in this section, couples who share the same cultural background can still have differences. Be curious by asking questions respectfully and with a sincere desire to understand.

2. **Validate your partner.** Now that you understand the purpose of your partner's boundary, express verbal acknowledgement of what they shared with you. As a reminder, validating statements sound like:

    - *"That makes sense."*
    - *"I want to understand. Tell me more about this."*
    - *"Sounds like it's frustrating for you."*
    - *"I'm starting to see how hard it can be for you when someone pushes that boundary."*
    - *"That has not been my experience in our culture; however, I want you to know I am here for you, and I understand this affects you."*
    - *"It sounds like you feel out of control when this happens. Am I getting it right?"*

    If you are having trouble validating your partner, it might be helpful to revisit the section on page 107.

3. **Share your concerns about the boundary.** Explain to your partner how their boundary impacts you or your ability to maintain

cultural practices that are important to you. What are you worried about happening? What do you hope for instead? Be mindful of sharing this as your perspective while still holding your partner's perspective in mind. You don't want to refute them in this part of the process as that directly negates the efforts you made in the previous step to validate them.

4. **Receive your partner's validation.** Hopefully, you and your partner are reading this book together, and your partner has also learned how to validate you. If this isn't the case, I encourage you to manage your expectations as your partner may not know how to validate you. However, you can try communicating your needs before you share your concerns in the previous step. You can say something like, *"I am hoping for an opportunity to explain my concerns fully and to receive some sort of acknowledgment from you to know you understand my perspective. Feeling understood is important to me. If you don't understand something I said, please ask me questions so I can clarify."*

5. **Negotiate what seems fair to both of you.** Now that both of you feel heard and understood, discuss what seems fair to both of you in the context of everything that was shared. Avoid getting into a me-against-you mentality. You are in a relationship together; therefore, what is important to your partner deserves sincere consideration from you. Focus on making this a win-win. Remember to lead the discussion with respect, compassion, and compromise. If the conversation becomes heated, make a decision to pause and regulate your emotions before continuing, as outlined in the steps on page 144.

The following is a list of questions you can ask each other or reflect upon during this discussion:

- How flexible is my/your boundary? How much can I/you tolerate before it affects our mental health?
- What might make something more tolerable for me/you?
- How much room is there to adjust my/your boundary to accommodate what is important to the other partner?
- What is fair to both of us in this situation?
- How can I support my partner's mental health better while also protecting my mental health?
- What boundaries and cultural practices can I/you re-evaluate now that we both understand each other better?
- Are there resources or support I/you can turn to within or outside our culture to help us manage differences in cultural practices and individual boundaries?
- Should we consider couple's therapy if we can't negotiate a boundary on our own?
- Am I open to working with a therapist so I can learn to be more supportive to my partner?
- Am I open to working with a therapist so I can heal the reason why I am maintaining a boundary strongly, even when I am aware of its negative impact on my partner and/or family members?

For some of you, the idea of establishing a boundary may seem next to impossible despite my recommendations. You may not see any way of setting a boundary without facing harsh consequences from your spouse, your parents, your in-laws, or from society for violating foundational cultural and religious expectations. You may have determined it is easier for you to accept relationships without healthy boundaries, even if it comes at the expense of your mental health. In other words, the risk of losing these relationships seems greater than the benefit of protecting your mental health. If this sounds like your struggle, you can consider the following options:

1. Learn how to establish healthy boundaries and figure out ways to mitigate the impact of the consequences.
2. Accept things as they are and find peace as you locate other ways of supporting your mental health.
3. Seek out and practice healthy coping skills to manage your mental health until you feel ready to establish boundaries.

Before I move on to the next section, I want to pause here and address a particular type of woman who may be reading this book. This woman resides in a part of the world where her rights are not recognized or supported and where women do not have the ability to speak out in ways that women in other parts of the world may have. For the woman who cannot safely advocate for her boundaries, I want to acknowledge how important your mental health and your personal safety is, including the mental health and safety of your children. While I do not have a solution to this challenge, I will restate and validate that your boundaries are worth respecting. *You* are worth respecting. And for all the women and mothers around the world, I want you to know violence is never acceptable. Every woman deserves to have a voice that is heard, respected, and understood no matter what part of the world she lives in, what culture she belongs to, or what relationship she finds herself in.

Boundaries with Family Members

Some of the hardest relationships to set boundaries in are those among family members. This is especially the case among individuals who grew up in families where either non-boundaries or unhealthy boundaries were modeled by adults. The reason it can be difficult to set boundaries with family members is often due to the roles different members of the family fall into from early on, and the expectation that these roles, the relationship dynamics, and behavioral patterns within the family system will remain unchanged.

Boundaries in family systems can be understood through the lens of structural family therapy, an approach developed by Salvadore Minuchin (1974). This type of psychotherapy analyzes family units, sub systems, hierarchies, boundaries, and triangulations. According to Minuchin, an integral part of a healthy family unit is the ability of members to maintain a sense of belonging to each other while also maintaining a sense of self. In other words, members of the family may largely share the same experiences, beliefs, traditions, and values, but they are also autonomous. This is where boundaries fit in.

Through the structural family therapy lens, setting boundaries can be tough with family members because of the underlying belief that change in one family member or one subsystem (example: sibling subsystem, parent subsystem, or a parent-child subsystem) can cause a ripple effect throughout the rest of the family unit. In other words, setting a boundary within one subsystem can destabilize the entire family unit. The destabilization is what can cause tension or conflict among family members because it can feel threatening to the unity or the sense of belonging. In this period of destabilization, the member who is establishing the boundary might experience pushback, or worse, be cut off from a particular member, subsystem, or the entire family.

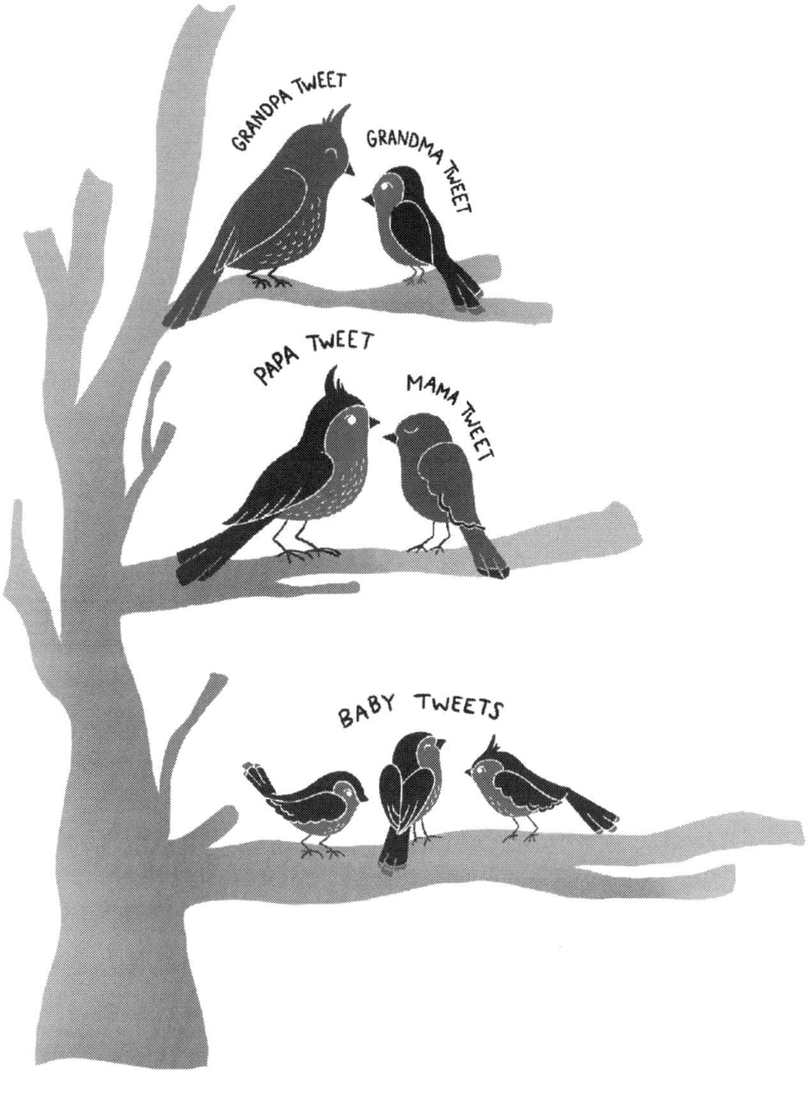
GRANDPA TWEET
GRANDMA TWEET
PAPA TWEET
MAMA TWEET
BABY TWEETS

Since establishing boundaries with family members can be challenging, I recommend clients to follow my four Cs method:

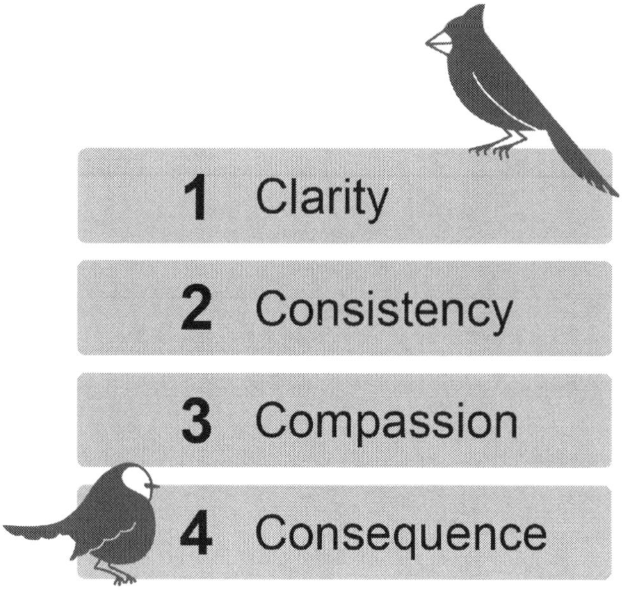
1 Clarity
2 Consistency
3 Compassion
4 Consequence

Setting boundaries in close relationships is more of a process rather than a single act. Sometimes, you may need to remind loved ones of your boundary a few times with consistency, clarity, and compassion. Your message should be simple and clear, focusing on you, and it should be the same message communicated a few times as gentle reminders until it sticks for the other person. The key to help the boundary stick is communicating and following through with consequence, that is, the action(s) you will take if you feel someone is ignoring, dismissing, or violating your boundary. A consequence is not meant as a threat or an ultimatum; rather, it is meant to convey how important your boundary is to you and what steps you're willing to take to respect your own boundary.

Here is an example of how you can use the Cs to communicate your boundary:

"I know you're so excited for the baby to arrive. I just feel uncomfortable when someone touches my belly. I prefer you ask me next time before doing it. And if you forget, no problem, I'll take a step back and remind you."

This is an example of an expectant mother who is learning to establish a physical boundary with a family member who repeatedly touches her belly without asking. The mother leads with compassion, acknowledging the family member's excitement. At the same time, she articulates her boundary firmly, using a few words to explain her feeling and her preference. She also communicates a consequence to help the family member understand how important the boundary is to her.

Depending on which family member or subsystem you are establishing your boundary with, it might be helpful to determine a few different ways you can communicate your boundary in case there is pushback. I will share an example of a new mother, Amelia, who is compassionately establishing a boundary with her mother-in-law, who visits several times a week:

"I am grateful for all the help you provided me these last few weeks. It would have been tough for me to do this without your support. I also value the memories you have created with Emma since her birth. And as I say this, I also want to share with you my struggles in figuring out a routine with her. She requires frequent naps and feedings, and I have come to learn that she responds better to structure and consistency. Creating a routine will also help me to have predictable times where I can focus on getting other things done around the house or get some rest. Going forward, how do you feel about coming over to help me with Emma once a week?"

This type of approach might not be safe to implement in all relationships; therefore, you will need to determine what feels safe to you. In Amelia's case, she knew that the best way to approach the boundary with her mother-in-law was through expressing appreciation and empathy. Thus, she checked in with her mother-in-law's feelings as she communicated her new boundary. The important thing to understand is that Amelia asked the question as a way of maintaining connection with her mother-in-law, and not with the intention of changing her boundary based on the response she received. Amelia was prepared to repeat the message in a gentle but firm way:

"I hear what you are saying and I can understand why you are feeling hurt. It makes sense because you have done so much to help me. Emma and I are grateful for this, and I appreciate you. At the same time, we both need some time alone together to settle into a good routine. Is there a day you prefer to come over? Emma will be so happy to see you every week."

As is demonstrated by Amelia's response, it might help to respond compassionately if you decide to ask a loved one how they feel about your boundary. You do not have to agree with what they say, but validating their feelings may soften their reaction to your boundary. If your family member does not seem to be responding well, you may decide it is best to keep it short and not inquire more about their feelings.

Be patient and kind with the process and try not to over-explain as that may complicate matters. Keep it simple and consistent. The family member may need time to process this new boundary and make sense of how it impacts them. They may be angry, hurt, or defensive at first, and they may even test the limits to see how far they can go with pushing the boundary. With simple, consistent, and compassionate messaging, the family member is more likely to come around to respecting your new boundary even if they don't understand it or agree with it. With time, they may realize it is not a threat but an attempt to establish a healthier relationship between the two of you.

When Boundaries Are Not Respected

Whenever you set a new boundary in a relationship, expect pushback. It is something the other person—be it your partner, a family member, an in-law, a co-worker, or a friend—does not expect. They are used to interacting with you a certain way. Now that you are teaching them what you are comfortable and not comfortable with, they will probably go through their own process of unlearning how they are used to interacting with you and learning to accept your new ways of interacting with them. This is the part that can take a little time and may require some patience on your part.

The pushback from your loved one might be their struggle in understanding your new boundary, or it may be an intentional act to test your boundary and see how firmly it holds. Whichever the case, it is important to remind your loved one that your boundary is important to you. You can do this by following through with a consequence, such as reminding them of the boundary, changing the topic, stepping away, or exiting the situation. This demonstrates your intention to maintain your boundary despite their pushback in order to safeguard your mental health.

Let's take a look at an example of how a couple can handle a situation with a family member who is not respectful of their boundary:

Sofia and Carlos, along with their three-year-old son and six-month-old daughter, temporarily moved into Carlos's parents' basement as they waited for their new house to be ready for them to move in. What was supposed to be a few months turned into over a year due to delays in construction because of the pandemic. Sofia found herself becoming increasingly agitated with her in-laws giving her son, Oscar, sugary snacks whenever he asked for one—which could be several times a day! Sofia had politely requested her in-laws a few times to limit his snacking—however, to no avail. She felt particularly frustrated when they would give him snacks right before dinner as it made mealtimes more difficult to manage. The frustration would build up into anger towards Oscar when he would refuse to eat dinner, complaining he wasn't hungry.

Each night, Sofia went to bed feeling guilty for being angry with her son when she knew it wasn't his fault for being full from snacking all day. The guilt was compounded with how bad she felt for not being able to give Oscar more time ever since her daughter was born. The guilt would lead to Sofia becoming harsh and unforgiving with herself. Feeling stuck for months in a toxic cycle of anger, guilt, and self-criticisms, Sofia leaned on Carlos for support. She explained to him how his parents were part of the reason for why she felt the way she did. Carlos expressed his understanding and asked Sofia how he could help her. Upon discussion, the couple agreed to set a clear boundary with the parents regarding snacks.

The couple approached the parents one night after the children were in bed. They explained to them how Oscar was skipping dinner most nights and why it was important to not give in to his demands for sugary snacks throughout the day, especially before meals. They requested the parents to limit it to one snack during the day and also provided them with alternative nutritious snacks for their son. The couple explained why this was important not only for their son's physical health but also for Sofia's mental health.

Carlos's father remained quiet, but his mother responded to all of this by becoming defensive. She exclaimed that she knew how to raise children, and that Sofia and Carlos were ungrateful for raising an issue over snacks instead of thanking them for their help. Carlos validated his mother, "You both have done so much to help us over this past year, and we understand this is coming across as ungrateful to you. We want to clarify what this is about: Oscar doesn't eat his dinner when he has had several snacks leading up to it. Dinnertime has become very difficult for both of us, especially for Sofia. She and I are asking for your help to make dinnertime easier for us by limiting snacks to one in the day."

Carlos's mother still seemed angry. Before she could respond, his father jumped in to say, "All right, all right, we get it. We will look after it." Knowing his parents well, Carlos expected his mother to continue giving sugary snacks to Oscar as many times as he asked and expected his father to remain quiet in order to avoid conflict with his wife. Thus, to demonstrate how important Sofia's mental health was to him, Carlos added, "Thank you for understanding, Dad. As grateful as I am to both of you for letting us live here and helping us out with the kids, I am also concerned about Sofia and Oscar. I want to make sure this doesn't continue being an issue going forward. If I notice Oscar still complaining about being full and refusing to eat dinner, I'll need to accompany him when he comes upstairs to you to manage his habit of snacking in the evenings."

Certain boundaries, when violated, may be more triggering for you than other boundaries. In this case, it is important for you to uphold them firmly, regardless of your partner or family member needing time to understand. For example, sexual boundaries are more triggering when they are violated than some of the other boundaries due to their vulnerable nature. Therefore, a sexual boundary is one that needs to be communicated explicitly and firmly, with an expectation for it to be respected right away. Your partner may have questions and want to understand you better, and while they may not fully understand at first, it will be vital for you to clearly communicate that you need them to respect your boundary.

Kristen and Alex welcomed their daughter nine months ago. Alex began to notice a change in Kristen in the last few months. She was no longer interested in sex, she seemed to be avoiding him at night, and she recoiled from him whenever he tried to show her physical affection. This left Alex feeling confused and hurt. He feared what was happening because physical affection and sexual intimacy was how the couple usually communicated their love to each other. It's what connected them the most. Alex became focused on trying to maintain this connection by approaching Kristen more frequently with physical affection and gestures of intimacy.

Kristen didn't understand what was happening herself. All she knew was that she wanted physical space from Alex. She was still breastfeeding and felt tied down to her daughter, who wanted to be in her mother's arms all day. Kristen began feeling hyper-vigilant and sensitive to Alex's physical proximity and touch. It made her skin crawl, and she felt agitated around him. Sometimes, she would snap at him, telling him to stop and to leave her alone.

Kristen would see the hurt on Alex's face, feel guilty, and become angry with herself. She even started feeling irritable with her daughter for always physically needing her in some way or another. It felt like her body couldn't catch a break, and sex was the furthest thing from her mind. Yet, Alex seemed to expect it even more from her. Because of her guilt, Kristen would sometimes give in and have sex instead of telling Alex how she really felt. After sex, Kristen would feel disgusted with herself for doing something she didn't feel comfortable with, and that started to build resentment inside of her towards Alex. With this resentment came even less desire to be touched by her partner during the day, even when it was something as sweet as a peck on her cheek before he went to work.

It became a vicious cycle, and Kristen decided to seek professional help. She worked with a therapist to help her understand what was going on inside of her. Soon, Kristen realized she was feeling completely "touched out" since having her baby. In other words, it overwhelmed her senses when anyone tried to touch her. For someone who typically felt very comfortable and looked forward to physical intimacy with her partner, this didn't make any sense to Kristen. How could she have a negative reaction to Alex giving her a kiss on the cheek?

With the help of her therapist, she came to understand how physical touch was no longer associated with feelings of love and affection for her. Instead, physical touch became associated with feelings of stress, anxiety, loss of freedom, frustration, and built-up resentment for Kristen as she felt she was the only one who could carry, hold, soothe, rock, and feed her daughter. This compounded with the feelings of guilt, disgust, and resentment that became associated with sex. As a result of all these underlying feelings, her body was now physiologically reacting to anticipating touch and being touched.

As Kristen began to make sense of what was happening, she decided it was important to establish new boundaries with Alex. She hoped this would not only improve her mental health but also her relationship. Sitting down with Alex one night, Kristen explained how she was feeling touched out, why that made her want to avoid him, her negative feelings towards sex, and how all of this was taking a toll on her mental health. She spoke with an open heart but remained respectful and compassionate. She remembered to use the tools for effective communication she'd learned in therapy. She welcomed Alex's questions with patience, knowing how this was something new for him and would require some time for him to understand.

Towards the end of the conversation, Kristen clearly, gently, and firmly communicated her new boundaries to Alex. The following is a dialogue between the couple:

Kristen:
"Alex, for the reasons I explained, I prefer we hang out, watch TV, have family time together, talk about our day… you know, just be with each other without any expectations of physical intimacy. Just for the time being. It would help me feel so much more comfortable and relaxed around you. And as for sex, I would like to be asked whether it is something I am in the mood for before you initiate it."

Alex:
"That seems a little unfair that I can't touch you. And touch is one thing, how can you tell me that you don't want us to have sex anymore? Doesn't that sound wrong to you?"

Kristen:
"I know it wouldn't be fair to ask you never to touch me. That wouldn't be normal for us. And I want us to go back to how we were before. What I am sharing with you is only meant for the time being while I figure out ways to cope better with being touched and needed all day."

Alex:
"How do I know this isn't forever? How do I know you will go back to normal and this wouldn't change us?"

Kristen:
"If I was in your shoes, I would be worried about the same thing. I can't speak about the future, but what I know is right now I am on-edge when I'm touched. I want to feel comfortable and relaxed around you like I always used to be. And for that reason, I prefer just hanging out together without the pressure of having to receive a hug or a kiss, you know?"

Alex:
"Okay, fine, but what about sex? You're saying you don't want to have sex either. I find that a bit extreme."

Kristen:
"On most days right now, I don't feel like having sex. And it stirs up a lot of negative feelings inside of me when I force myself to go along with it. What I prefer is you ask me instead of assuming that it's what I want. Going forward, I'm no longer going to force myself to have sex if I am not feeling okay about it. It's doing more harm than good for me and our relationship. And if I feel like you're forgetting or that I'm being pushed, I will remind you."

Alex remained quiet, looking into the distance with a frown on his face. Kristen spoke her next words carefully, with compassion: *"Alex, I know this is a lot to take in. I don't normally set boundaries like this with you, especially around sex, but this is to prevent myself from spiraling into a worse place in our relationship. I want to feel close and connected to you. I am requesting that we find different ways to connect right now while I learn to cope better with my feelings around being touched and having sex."*

Alex:
"I need some time to think about what you said. It's a lot to process right now."

Kristen:
"I understand. We can talk about this again once you have had some time to think about it."

The exchange between Kristen and Alex was a difficult conversation. However, with effective communication skills such as validation, vulnerability, compassion, respect, clarity, and consistency to express her new boundaries, Kristen was able to manage the conversation well. Kristen also ended the conversation knowing this wasn't the last time the couple would talk about it. However, in spite of the time Alex needed to understand these new boundaries, she made it explicitly clear to him that she would no longer force herself to engage in sex if her body wasn't feeling open to it.

If you find yourself in a relationship that does not respect your boundaries despite clear and consistent messaging, you have a few choices to make. You can:

1. Have an open conversation with your loved one(s) about your concerns and feelings when your boundaries are not respected to see if that makes a difference.
2. Learn to increase your distress tolerance as a way of coping. This can be done by:
   - Learning to manage your expectations about whether your boundary will be respected
   - Finding a support system, such as leaning on your spouse for comfort when you are around a loved one who ignores your boundaries
   - Developing regulation skills to manage your emotions and reactions to the offending family member
   - Going to therapy to learn coping skills and how to manage the offending family member more effectively
3. Distance yourself from the relationship, if possible.
4. Make the difficult decision to end the relationship, if possible.

These choices are the same whether with your partner, parents, siblings, in-laws, friends, or co-workers. Learning to set boundaries can be a challenging experience, and one that requires courage. When you are establishing new boundaries, go in with the expectation that there will be pushback so you are not surprised if it happens. Remember that people may not understand you, and they may react negatively to your boundary. Remind yourself that your loved one(s) are learning something new about you, and they may need some time to adjust to this change. Finally, know that you have the ability to choose and decide what you would like to do if your loved one(s) don't respect your boundaries.

Managing Expectations of Yourself

An important part of self-care is learning to manage expectations of yourself as a parent. Sometimes, these expectations are set by others, such as your spouse, family, or society. Other times, they are set on you by no one other than yourself! These expectations are often more heavily felt by the primary parent, usually the mother. Mothers feel the responsibility of the development and nourishment of their child from the moment they conceive: nourishing their baby in the womb, carrying their baby to full term, birthing their baby safely, breastfeeding, comforting, soothing, and beyond.

If the expectations are not met, whether they are set by herself or by someone else, it leaves many mothers feeling like they are failing the standards of motherhood because of the unconscious belief that you are a "good" mother only if you meet these standards. Therefore, meeting these expectations becomes synonymous with being a "good" mother. For some, this inherently means they are a "bad" mother if they struggle to meet these expectations. These mothers come to believe they are not worthy or capable of being a mother. Working hard to meet these expectations can create self-doubts, leaving mothers feeling disappointed in themselves, questioning their capabilities, feeling anxious and depressed, and experiencing burnout.

Expectations about self as a parent also come from mental images which new parents hold on to subconsciously. These images are about what it is like to be a "good" parent. For example, if you are expecting a baby while reading this book, think about what images and words come to mind when you imagine yourself as a parent. If you have already had your baby, think about what images and words came to your mind when you used to imagine yourself as a parent versus how you are as a parent now. Both mothers and fathers have subconscious mental images of what they think being a good parent would be like. These images can be informed by how your parents were when you were a child, other parents in your familial or social circle, movies, books, social media, and societal, cultural, and religious expectations of what it is to be a "good" parent.

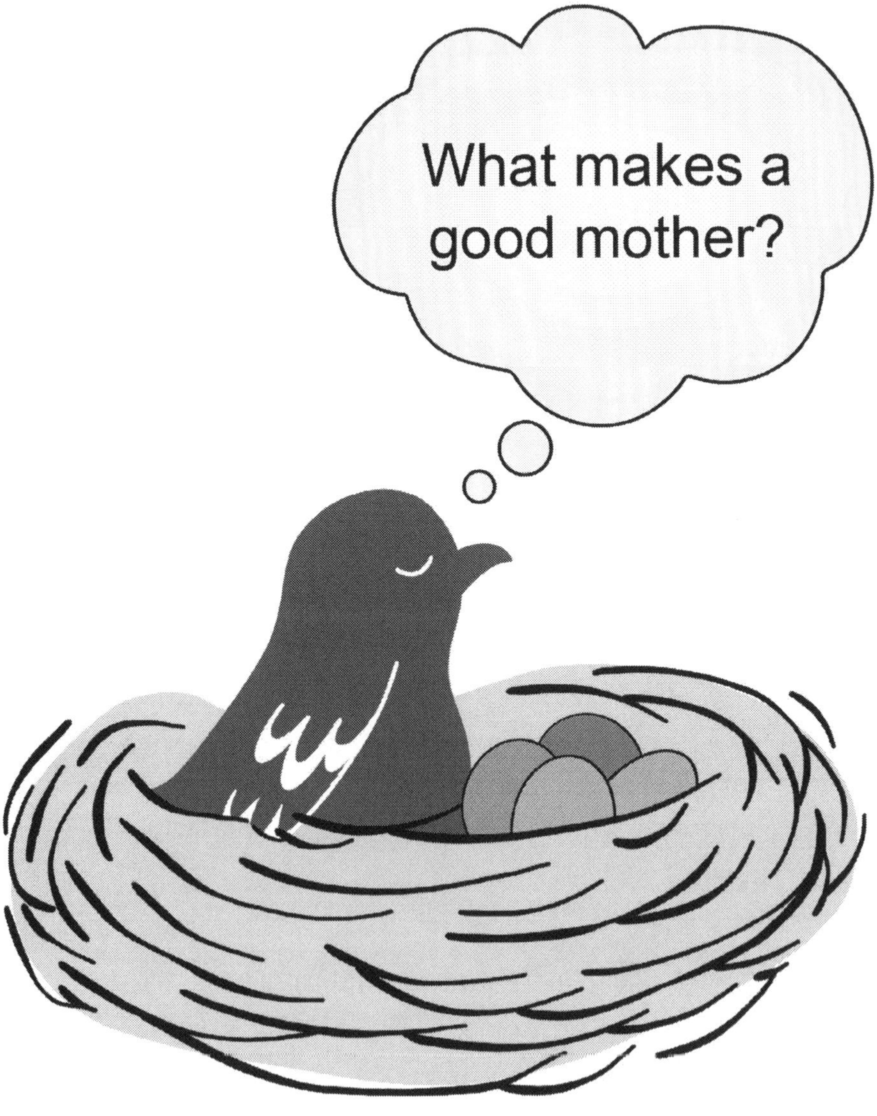
What makes a good mother?

Having these subconscious mental images is not a bad thing. However, it can impact your mental health if you experience tension between who you are as a parent versus the image you had in your mind. This internal tension (which can be outside of your conscious awareness) can be explained by the Maternal Postpartum Role Collapse Theory (Amankwaa, 2005). This theory is divided into three components: role stress, role strain, and role collapse.

Role stress is explained as the worries mothers experience in the postpartum period, such as questioning their capabilities as a parent. Role strain is described as the emotional response mothers experience in response to the role stress, such as anger, guilt, frustration, disappointment, or shame. With enough of a strain, mothers can experience role collapse when they find the strain too difficult to cope with. A mother experiencing a collapse might fall into postpartum depression (Amankwaa, 2005). I would argue this theory can be expanded to include both mothers and fathers; thus, I will refer to this as parental role collapse.

Parental Role Collapse

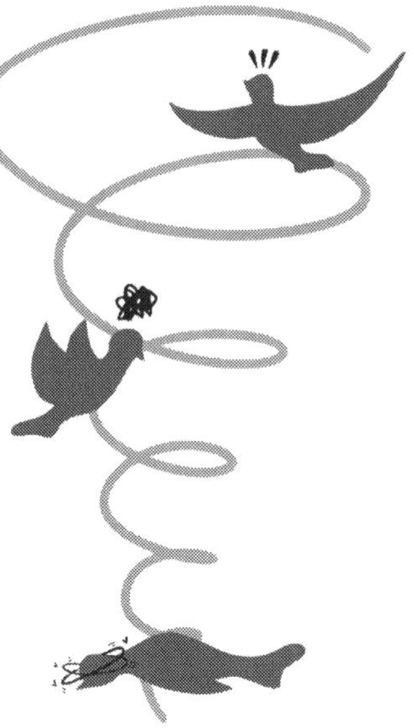

Role Stress
Thoughts about a postpartum stressor

Role Strain
Emotional response incited by the thoughts towards the stressor

Role Collapse
Maladaptive behavioral response to cope with the emotions

I experienced role stress after each of my children were born as I worried about my inability to breastfeed them successfully. It didn't take long for me to experience strain as my worries turned into feelings of frustration, disappointment, and guilt. In retrospect, a big aspect of my mental image of a "good" mother included happy, loving, and bonding experiences of breastfeeding my children. Since reality was different each time from this subconscious image, I started to lose confidence in myself as a mother during both my breastfeeding experiences. Eventually, I headed towards collapse.

Within days of my son's birth, I began to dread feeding him. My poor baby would struggle to latch, screaming and crying out of hunger. This would bring up feelings of confusion, tears, guilt, and frustration inside of me. When my son and I finally got the hang of breastfeeding and we both started to enjoy it—which was around three months postpartum—I rapidly began to lose my supply. At first, I felt confused. How could this be? We were finally enjoying our time together, with him snuggled up in my arms and me staring into his peaceful and drowsy face as he fed comfortably. This was the magical experience I had been yearning for all those times he screamed and cried in my arms as I desperately tried to figure out how to help him latch. How could this magical time come to an end? It felt like a cruel joke.

By the fourth month, when I was barely producing any milk, I panicked. I started to research all the ways I could get my supply back up. Then I felt angry. I don't know who I was angry with. But I was angry because it felt so unfair! Eventually I felt sad and hopeless because this was out of my control. I remember feeling a sense of doom for a few days when it was coming to an end. And just like that, within two weeks, I went from being able to somewhat breastfeed my son to having nothing left to offer him. At 4.5 months postpartum, this shattered me. I still remember the very last time I fed him—and I knew at the time this was the last time. I remember looking at his face in my arms as he fed, trying to memorize every detail of it. It's as if I was taking a photograph with my mind so I could hold on to the memory of this moment forever. It's strange how raw and intense emotions can feel sometimes.

Once my supply was completely finished, I felt I was grieving. I had my son in my arms, yet I felt I no longer shared the same relationship with him. The nine months I carried him and the four months I breastfed him, only I could give him what he needed. Only I could carry him, nourish him, and comfort him. But when I lost my ability to feed him, I was no longer the only person he needed. Now anyone could feed him from the bottle. Now anyone could give him the comfort he needed. That part of the special relationship between him and I was gone. Forever.

On a rational level, I know this isn't true. I know my son will continue to need me in different ways. But on an emotional level, there was nothing that felt as true as what I was feeling in those days. What made matters worse is that none of it fit within my mental image of what I thought being a mother and caring for my child looks like. In other words, I wasn't meeting the standards of motherhood which were preconceived in my mind.

I had a very different experience when my daughter was born, and unfortunately, it came with its own set of challenges. In many ways, my breastfeeding journey with my daughter was worse than it was with my son. Once again, none of the difficulties I experienced fit the mental image in my mind of what it is like to be a mother.

To give context, my daughter would not breastfeed, and she would refuse the bottle. I felt helpless for months. Because she wouldn't breastfeed for more than two or three minutes at a time, I had an extremely low supply. I also tried everything under the sun to get her to take the bottle—but she refused fervently. My husband and I would try for hours, but she would scream at the top of her lungs, crying the entire time without taking a single sip of milk. By the time my daughter was three months old, she had dropped to the third percentile on the weight curve, which seemed alarmingly low. The stress of trying to feed our daughter also caused friction between my husband and I in the initial weeks since her birth. To name all the emotions, I felt lost, confused, helpless, scared, angry, anxious, exhausted, and overwhelmed. What's worse, having this endless stream of feelings made me feel like a bad mother, and I started disliking myself.

To give you the full picture, I should also mention this was happening at the start of the COVID-19 pandemic. When the pandemic began, I was in my final month of pregnancy and gave birth during a time when no one understood what was happening in the world or what to expect. We were living in complete isolation and uncertainty for months with a newborn and a toddler at home. All of this culminated into me developing postpartum anxiety. At the time, I did not have the clarity of mind to recognize any of this.

It was not until six months postpartum that I felt my worst and decided to see my therapist. A lot of my issues stemmed from the feelings of anger and hatred I felt towards myself for not being a better mother and a better wife. I subconsciously compared myself to the images I had in my mind of what a good mother and a good wife is, not recognizing those images did not take any of the following into account: how incredibly challenging it was both physically and mentally to get my daughter to feed from me, my daughter's refusal to drink milk from the bottle, her inability to gain adequate weight for several months after birth, a global pandemic, being locked down for months with no end in sight, isolation from friends and family, caring for a toddler and a newborn 24/7 with no outside support due to the pandemic, feelings of disconnect from my spouse, uncertainties and anxiety from the unknowns of the time, lack of freedom to live life as I once knew, and so much more.

Looking back now, I am able to say I was not fair to myself when I compared myself to images of what it is like to be a wife and a mother of two small children in a peachy world. In reality, the world was far from peachy. And my life felt like a mess. I wish at the time I'd had the clarity of mind to manage my expectations of myself as a mother, as a wife, and as a person. I am grateful, however, that with the help of therapy, I was eventually able to understand what I was experiencing and feel compassion towards myself. Being able to increase self-compassion and manage expectations of myself created a significantly positive shift in my mental health because it allowed me to accept who I was, how I was, and what I was experiencing without hating myself.

As part of my work in therapy, I also came to realize I not only needed to manage my own expectations, but I also needed to manage other people's expectations of me. To illustrate how I did this, I will share the example of the days when I was struggling to breastfeed my son as a new mother:

About four weeks after giving birth to my son, I realized my inability to breastfeed him successfully was taking a toll on my physical and mental health, and I needed to do something about it. I decided to educate myself better on the topic of breastfeeding, not from the medical perspective, but from the perspective of other moms. As I mentioned in Chapter 1, I spent each waking moment at night (and there were many, many waking moments with my son) reading questions, comments, and stories from mothers around the world who shared similar, or worse breastfeeding experiences than mine. And many mothers, including myself, shared a few things in common: we felt helpless, angry, incapable, and guilty. I started to reflect on why we were feeling this way. If breastfeeding did not come as naturally to every mother as is mistakenly assumed, then why do we carry so many self-doubts? Who is making us doubt ourselves as mothers?

As I reflected on this, I came to the following conclusions about where the expectations were coming from which drove my inner turmoil on the experience of breastfeeding as a new mother:

1. I didn't want to disappoint my husband because he expected me to breastfeed our son. He was well-intentioned and there was no force involved, yet I felt the weight of the expectation clearly.
2. I didn't want to deprive my son of what I understood to be his right, an expectation I felt through cultural and religious messaging.
3. I was subconsciously influenced by the expectation that a mother should feel pride and honor in being able to feed her child, a message that is prevalent across societies, cultures, and religions. This was further confirmed by subliminal messaging from family members who innocently shared their experiences of breastfeeding as mothers.
4. I was strongly influenced by the widely held expectation that a mother should feed her child breast milk because it is important to the nourishment and development of a healthy baby. Understandably, this expectation is perpetuated by medical experts,

lactation experts, blogs and articles on the Internet, mothers on social media, societies at large, cultures, and religions.

5. Both my husband and I expected me to give our son a healthy, clean start to life without depending on formula unnecessarily.

By identifying these sources of expectations, I became conscious of what was weighing me down. Gaining this self-awareness helped me to decide whose expectations mattered most to me, and whether those expectations were fair in terms of my limitations. My limitations did not diminish my strengths and capabilities as a mother—a realization that took me some time to appreciate. Ultimately, I came to decide that besides my husband's expectations of me as a mother, my own expectations mattered the most to me. Thus, I was able to adjust my expectations from a place of self-awareness, and I made my decisions around breastfeeding accordingly.

I decided that feeding my son breast milk was important to me, not breastfeeding. Thus, I began pumping and gave him breastmilk through the bottle any time he struggled to latch. To set myself up for success, I created a pump schedule so I could ensure there was always breast milk ready to go. I decided to continue giving breastfeeding a chance, without the pressures caused by external expectations. If he latched, great! If he didn't, that was okay. I also held him each time with intention, reminding myself that the magical bonding experience didn't only need to happen during breastfeeding. And during the times he was able to breastfeed, I soaked in the feeling of love, gratitude, comfort, and joy.

I also researched formula brands and felt confident in the ingredients of one particular brand that was closest to breastmilk. I then began introducing it to my son right away without guilt or hesitation. Aside from making these adjustments to my expectations, I lovingly and intentionally gave myself this affirmation: *I will do the best I can every day, and I recognize that my best will look different each day.*

Since my husband's expectations mattered to me, I asked him questions to understand where his expectations of me were coming from. I learned his expectation around breastfeeding stemmed from concerns of my son's healthy development, which were the same concerns as mine. When I recognized we had similar concerns, I kept him informed of all my formula research. As we began having vulnerable conversations around the topic of breastfeeding, we began understanding each other better and realizing we both needed to adjust our expectations of me as a mother.

The process of recognizing and adjusting expectations is not a one-time thing. It is an ongoing conversation with yourself and your partner. It is also a conversation that may need to happen each time you have another child. I thought I had it tough trying to breastfeed my son. As it turned out, I had it even tougher with my daughter. This required new realizations and new adjustments to expectations of myself as a mother.

As you consider your self-care, I encourage you to identify any unmanaged expectations. Whether you are the mother or the father, here is a list of questions you can reflect on to help you begin:

- When I am experiencing a feeling repeatedly, such as anger, anxiety or guilt, what thoughts are associated with these feelings?
- Which thoughts have the words *should* or *should not* in them (indicates an expectation)?
- Where are these expectations coming from? Who told me to think this way?
- What impact are these expectations having on me, on my relationship with my partner, and on my relationship with my child?

- What purpose are these expectations serving in my life? Are they helping me or harming me?
- Do I want to continue trying to meet these expectations?
- What would I say to a friend who is trying to meet the same expectations?
- What can I say to myself? What do I need to remind myself of?
- If I'm struggling to manage these expectations, what can help me? Will it help to talk to another young parent? Will it help to educate myself better on a topic? Will it help to reassess which values are important to me? Do I need to work through some things with the help of a professional?

Managing Expectations of Your Partner

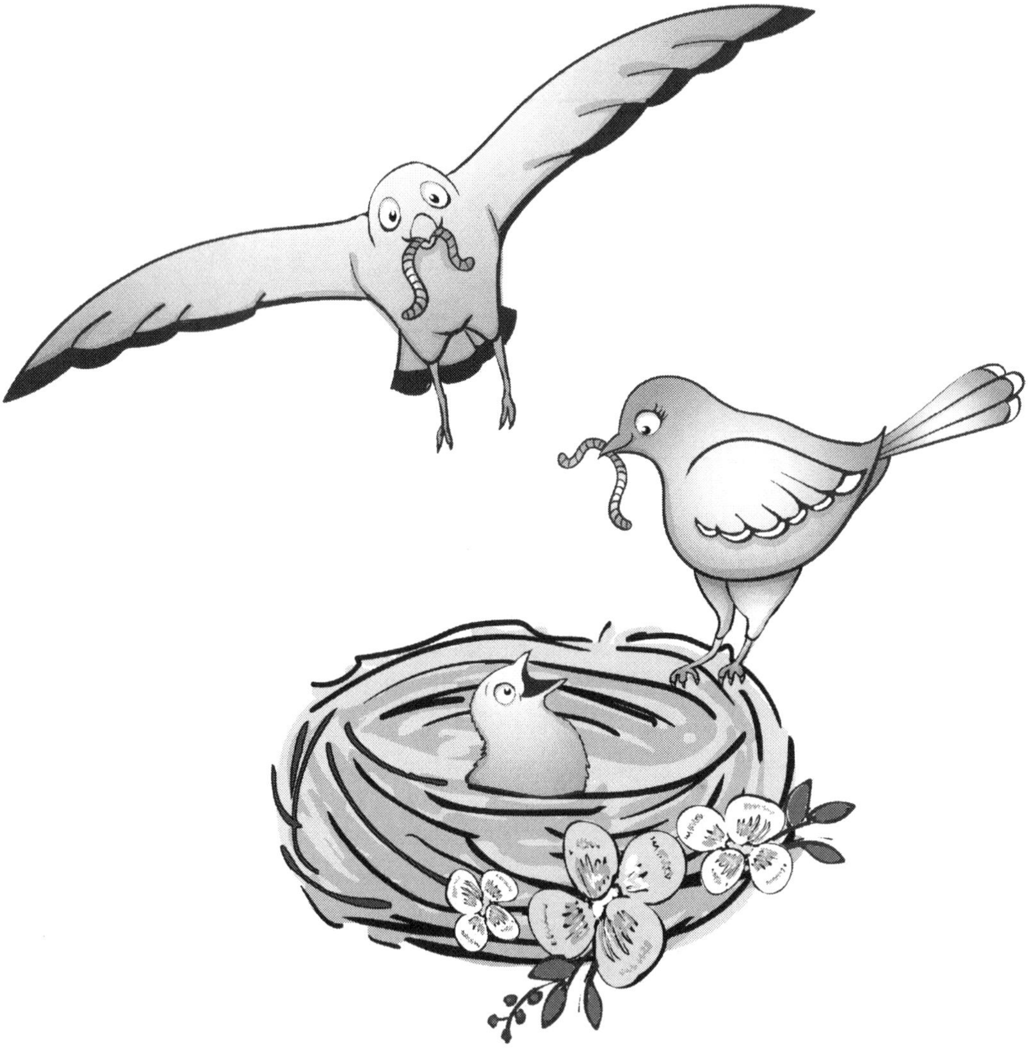

Equally important to your self-care, and to your partner's mental health, is learning to manage your expectations of your partner. Similar to how you experience the impact of conscious or unconscious expectations, so does your partner. If you are having trouble identifying what expectations you have of your partner, follow the similar process mentioned above to determine what you think your partner *should* or *should not* be doing. These expectations can be about them as a partner and/or as a parent. Once you are able to identify the expectations you hold of your partner, ask yourself the same set of questions as the ones listed at the end of the previous section.

Additionally, ask yourself: Have I communicated my expectations to my partner, or do I assume they know?

This question might be the most important question to ask yourself once you determine what type of expectations you have of your partner. Couples often create traps for their relationship by making assumptions about what their partner *should* already know or *should* be doing. While it is possible for two partners to become intuitive about each other after being in a relationship long enough, neither partner can be confident with one hundred percent accuracy that their assumptions are correct. With time and new experiences, people can change. Thoughts, opinions, feelings, perceptions, needs, likes, dislikes, and behaviors are all susceptible to change as an individual evolves over time. Therefore, your assumption about your partner can be accurate within one season of your relationship but inaccurate during a different season. This makes assumptions an unreliable tool in relationships. Finally, it is important to remember that even if you and your partner know each other intimately, you don't quite know each other yet as parents.

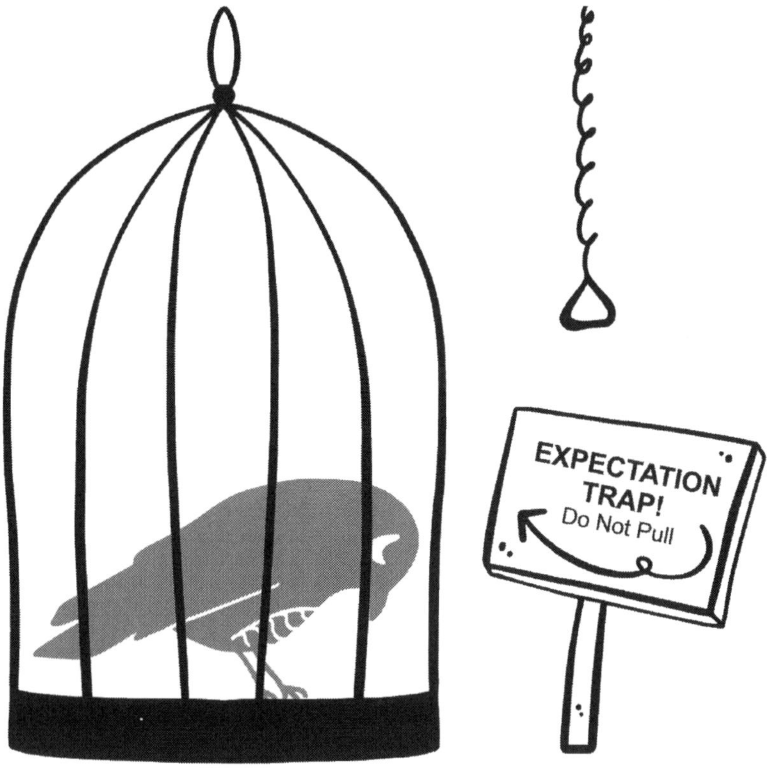
EXPECTATION
TRAP!
Do Not Pull

You can avoid making assumptions by simply communicating your expectations to each other. Engage in an open-ended discussion where you both share what you expect of each other as partners and as co-parents. Avoid criticisms, blaming, and other forms of harshness. Instead, approach each other with mutual respect, curiosity, and compassion as you communicate your expectation(s) as a request, not a demand. It might help you to review the sections on identifying emotional needs and building and maintaining emotional connection in Chapter 2 to help you phrase your expectations as requests.

When you engage in this discussion, also share with each other where your expectations come from and reflect on how these expectations impact both of you individually, as a couple, and as parents. This will help both of you gain new perspectives, understand each other better, and increase compassion. Finally, be open to reevaluating and adjusting your expectations as you learn about and understand each other better.

Conversations about expectations should occur periodically as you continue your evolution as parents to your child(ren) and partners to each other. To demonstrate how you can have this conversation, I will share the story of Sarah and Ahmad, a couple in their 30s who welcomed a baby boy in the second year of their marriage. Sarah is a stay-at-home mother, and Ahmad owns an auto repair business with long hours on the job.

Given his upbringing in a family with traditional gender role expressions, Ahmad's expectation of himself as the husband is he should be the one to shoulder all the financial burden of the family. He expects himself to be the breadwinner and work as much as possible to provide financial comfort for his wife and his child. Additionally, he expects his wife will do most of the childcare and household work.

Sarah's resentment towards her husband grows as the parenting and household load falls mainly on her shoulders since the birth of their son. Sarah's expectations about a marriage revolve around an equal share of roles where both husband and wife contribute to the finances, the household, and the care of children. This is what was modeled to Sarah in her family where she grew up watching her mother and father share responsibilities equally on all fronts.

The following is a conversation where the couple identifies and explores their expectations of each other:

Sarah:
"I realize I have been angry with you ever since Idris has been born because I feel like I am doing everything on my own while you are working. I feel exhausted taking care of Idris and everything else around the house."

Ahmad:
"I have noticed the anger but I don't understand where it comes from…"

Sarah:
"The anger comes from the fact that you don't help me enough. Before Idris was born, I imagined all the ways in which we were going to do things together, not only as husband and wife but as parents too. I imagined us as a team. But since he's been born, I feel like everything from childcare to housework is on my plate while you're away working nearly every day of the week. We don't do things together anymore. It feels like we are living separate lives."

Ahmad:
"I see it differently. I think we make a great team because I make sure you and Idris have a comfortable life free of financial stress, and you take care of him and our home. We both take care of different things and we both do it well."

Sarah:
"I know you work hard to make sure we have a comfortable life. However, it isn't your job alone to provide for us. You know well enough that I enjoy working and I plan to go back to work once he is a bit older. I also don't want you working so hard that you miss out on us being together as a family. More than financial comfort, what matters to me is your involvement in our life and our home. I want us to be a family unit with overlapping roles and responsibilities instead of living separate lives."

Ahmad:
"I guess we have different expectations of what I should be doing."

Sarah:
"I think we do. And as I'm talking about this, I'm realizing my expectation of what my husband would do comes from watching my dad around the house when I was growing up. I remember always seeing him helping my mom around the house and spending time with us on the weekends despite having a demanding job. He'd work late hours but, somehow, we

always felt his presence around us and he made it a point to spend a lot of time with us on weekends. I am realizing that I am expecting you to be the same way but I never shared this with you. I just assumed you will be the same way as my dad was to our family."

Ahmad:
"I definitely didn't know you expected this of me. I understand your dad helped your mom around the house. And I know I don't do that, but I do help watch Idris when I come home from work to give you a break. I thought I was showing my support to you by helping out in that way."

Sarah:
"Ahmad, you are not a babysitter giving me a break. You are his father and it is your role as a parent to spend time with your son. Maybe you have different expectations of what your role is as a father, but this is what my expectation is of you. And this is very important to me. I want Idris to remember having his dad around in his life the way I remember both my parents being around when I was growing up."

Ahmad remained silent for a few moments, looking like he's angry but holding back his words.Sarah picked up on this and asked him what was going on.

Ahmad:
"I'm starting to feel angry and I don't want to say something I regret. Give me a minute."

As Ahmad regulated his anger, Sarah quietly sat next to him in support. Once he felt calm enough to choose his words, Ahmad responded:

Ahmad:
"It's hurtful to hear you say I'm not around for my son when I'm working so hard to make sure he has a good life. It makes me feel like I am not a good father."

Sarah:
"You are such a good father and husband in many ways! I don't think I have shared how grateful I am to you for making sure every day, without fail, you give me a much needed break by watching Idris after work. It is such a big help, Ahmad. And both Idris and I are lucky to have you in our lives. You are working so hard to provide for our comfort and

well-being and I don't think I have been very good at sharing things like this with you."

Ahmad:
"That is the first time I am hearing you acknowledge my hard work, you know. And it feels nice for a change to be told I'm doing something right."

Sarah:
"I wish I was able to share more with you how I really feel. The reason why I probably haven't thought to thank you before is because my anger builds up by the time you come home. I am overwhelmed and on edge from doing things around the house while also looking after Idris all day. I am realizing now that my anger towards you isn't fair. I have been expecting you to help me around the house and be physically present more with us as a family the way my Dad was. This expectation is unfair, especially since I am not communicating it to you."

Ahmad:
"It is also unfair because I am a different person and we have very different financial circumstances than your family did when you were growing up."

Sarah:
"Yes, that is true."

Ahmad:
"Thank you for acknowledging all of this. I have really been struggling since Idris has been born. I feel like I can't get anything right and work is the only place I feel like I am succeeding. Maybe that's why I also haven't been around as much… and, you know, as you're telling me about your parents, I also probably haven't been around at home because I grew up in a household where Mom was always around taking care of things and Dad was always away working long hours and weekends to keep his business afloat. I never saw him help around the house, honestly, not once. I think I had the same expectation of us as a couple: I will work, and you will look after our children and our home."

Sarah:
"It's interesting how we both had such different expectations around what our roles will be after having children. I'm glad we are talking about this. It's helping me understand you better and why you haven't been helping me around the house."

Ahmad:
"Same. So what do we do from here? I want to be around more to help and be involved as a family unit but I also need a more supportive wife... you know, someone who is building me up instead of tearing me down."

Sarah:
"Can you help me understand what you mean by that? How do I tear you down?"

Ahmad:
"I just feel like I can't do anything right around you... like I am doing something wrong in your eyes. Or something I should be doing better."

Sarah:
"Yeah, I think I know what you mean. I do pick on you a lot when you are around. I am home with Idris all day so I just feel like I have a better way of doing things and I expect you to do it my way. But that's not fair to you. I bet it's annoying, huh?"

Ahmad:
"You have no idea! I'll get better at doing things a certain way with Idris as I spend more time around him but until then, I need some space and patience from you to let me figure it out."

Sarah:
"I will work on this. I miss having you around, Ahmad..."

Ahmad:
"I know, I miss being around you guys too. What can I do to be more helpful and involved?"

Sarah:
"I would find it helpful if you can take on some house chores so I don't feel overwhelmed from trying to do everything on my own. And, also, it would be nice to spend some time together at least on weekends as a family."

Ahmad:
"I recognize how important it is, not only for you but also for me, to spend time with our son. I will figure out a way to make this happen more frequently. As for house chores, I am not sure how I will balance that with work, but I am willing to try now that I hear how overwhelmed you have been. What kinds of things did you need help with around the house?"

Sarah:
"Let me give that some thought and get back to you. I understand from your perspective that it's important for you to work hard and provide for our family. And I don't want to pile things on your plate because I also see how tired you are when you come home from work. Maybe we can rethink our expectations of each other and let one another know more clearly what we need help with?"

Ahmad:
"That's fair. Let's give this some thought and talk about it this weekend."

Sarah and Ahmad communicated their expectations to each other after they realized they were experiencing tension and dissatisfaction in their relationship. However, I recommend sharing your expectations before your baby arrives. If you are expecting a child, now would be a great time to start reflecting on what mental images and expectations you have of yourself and each other, as a couple and as co-parents. Remember to communicate these expectations as requests, keeping yourself open to the idea of reevaluating and adjusting your expectations after talking to your partner and understanding them better. Like Sarah and Ahmad, work together as a team to discuss what is important to each of you, be respectful and kind, find common ground, and create a framework of shared meaning in your relationship.

You may need to revisit this conversation as you progress in your pregnancy and after your baby is born. With time, change, and new experiences, new expectations might develop or old expectations might resurface. It is especially important to revisit this conversation if you begin to feel any conflict or dissatisfaction in your relationship due to unmet expectations.

If you are still struggling to identify what expectations you have of each other, here is an introspective exercise which both of you can do separately and reflect upon together as a couple: In the house illustration, label each quadrant to represent different parts of your home, such as your bedroom, nursery, laundry room, kitchen, bathroom, and family room. Next, list out all the expectations you have of your partner in each of those rooms. Outside of the outline of the house, list out any expectations related to outside of your home. This can include yard work, grocery runs, daycare pick-ups and drop-offs, and so on.

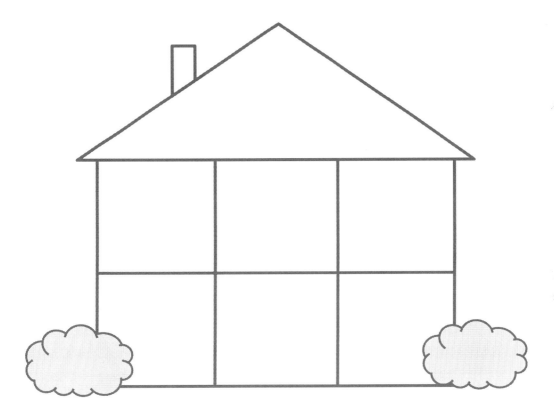

As I bring this section to a close, I want to remind you that experiencing tension, resentment, and anger in your relationship are all signposts pointing you in a direction that requires some attention, support, and perhaps healing. It's completely normal to experience negative emotions towards your partner and your relationship as you enter the learning curve of becoming parents and co-parents—whether for the first time, second time, or beyond. However, this awareness also needs to come with the understanding that it is up to you to communicate what you are thinking, feeling, and experiencing in a manner that is clear, kind, and respectful. Your partner is not a mind reader. They will not know or understand unless you let them know and help them understand you better using healthy communication.

In the empty talk bubble, script out how you might start a conversation with your partner around an unmet expectation which is causing tension in your relationship. For example, you may write something like, *"Honey, can I speak to you about some challenges I've been dealing with concerning chores around the house? I am feeling upset and somewhat abandoned in having to do everything myself. And I realize I am feeling this way because I have been expecting certain things from you without actually telling you directly. Are you open to talking about this right now? And if not, when is a good time for you?"*

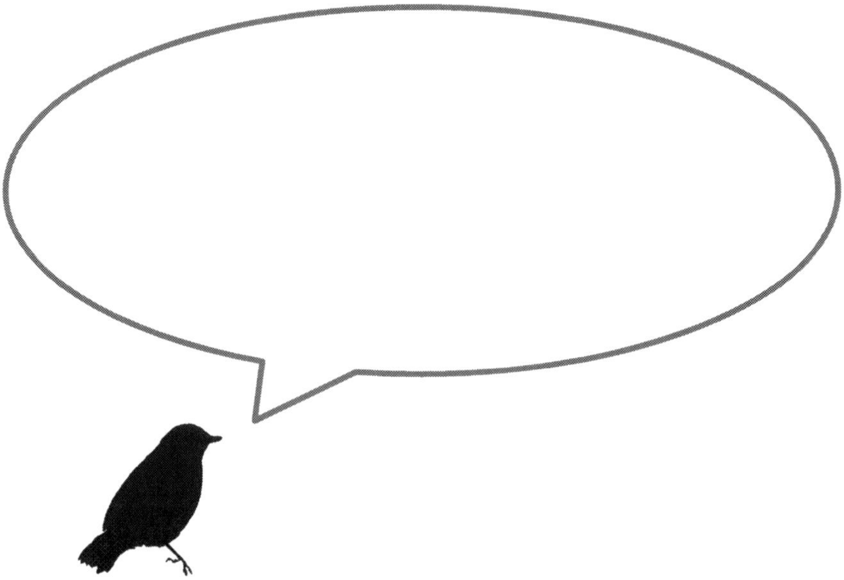

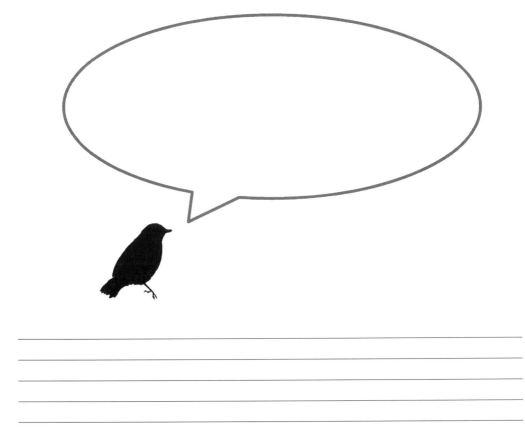

Self-Care Plan

If you are an expecting mother reading this book, I urge you to consider creating a self-care plan which you can turn to whenever you need additional support, now or after birth. In fact, it can be beneficial for both you and your partner to chalk out a rough plan which takes into account both people's needs. If you have already welcomed your baby, it is never too late to plan your self-care. If possible, take a few minutes right now and use the tips I provide in this section to create a plan so you are ready to implement it right away, or as soon as you're ready. Having a self-care plan helps you recognize forms of support in the right places with the right people, while helping you validate your needs, manage your expectations, feel prepared, and make stressors more manageable.

The plan should be clear, realistic, and achievable. To help you get started, here are some guidelines you can use to plan your self-care:

1. **What do you need help with?**

    - List out all the ways your **body** needs support during pregnancy or after birth. For example, your body may need sleep, rest in bed for recovery, a shower, a walk, a break from breastfeeding, help with physically demanding chores and errands, and physiotherapy. If this is your second pregnancy, you may need additional support from your partner or a family member to help with the care of your firstborn. This can include help with lifting your toddler in and out of their crib if you are advanced in your pregnancy, help with giving your toddler a bath if you are recovering from surgery, and help with babysitting so you can attend to your medical and physical care appointments.

    - List out all the ways your **mind** needs support during

pregnancy or after birth. For example, your mind may need self-compassion, affirmations, time alone to rest and rejuvenate, time with your partner to reconnect, a plan to visit a friend without your baby, support from your therapist, emotional regulation, planning meals for the week ahead of time so you feel less stressed, better time management, and some retail therapy to help build confidence in your new postpartum body.

2. **Who can you ask for help?**

Who is the best person to ask for help for each of the items you need support with? When answering this question, the key is to identify the person who is *naturally inclined* to support you in the way you need. For example, let's say you recognize your need for reassurance from a loved one on difficult days. Perhaps your partner is not always good at providing reassurance. Think of someone else in your circle who naturally tends to reassure you when you turn to them. It can be your mother, a friend who has gone through similar experiences, or someone in your community support group for new mothers.

3. **How can you ask for help?**

Regardless of who you have listed as a source of support in your self-care plan, I recommend communicating it to the person(s) ahead of time as a courtesy. More importantly, please remember it is unfair to expect your partner, or anyone else, to support you in the manner you are looking for without sharing your expectations beforehand.

The following is a dialogue between a couple, Tina and Jacob. Tina gave birth a couple of weeks ago to their daughter, Eva. Her husband, Jacob, works from home at a company he has been with for a few years, which allows him flexibility to help his wife during work hours. In this dialogue, Tina shares her care plan with Jacob and asks for his support. Here is how the couple engaged in this conversation:

TINA:
Jacob, I have created a self-care plan and I wanted to share it with you. Is now a good time?

JACOB:
Yeah, I am free right now. What is a self-care plan?

TINA:
It is something new I have learnt about. The idea is to make sure I have a plan in place to recognize when I need help with something and know who to turn to for support. This will help me take care of my mind and body so I can continue to do well in my role as a mother.

JACOB:
Sounds like a good idea. So what did you want to share?

TINA:
It has been 2 weeks since Eva has been born and my back and neck are really starting to ache from all the breastfeeding. I still want to keep it up as much as possible, but I'm wondering if I can lean on you to step in and bottle feed her when I ask for the help? That way, I can use the time to lay down and stretch my back for a few minutes.

JACOB:
Sure, I'd love to help! I'm jealous of all the cuddle time you two get with each other!

TINA:
Awesome, thank you! What's the best way I can let you know that I need the help?

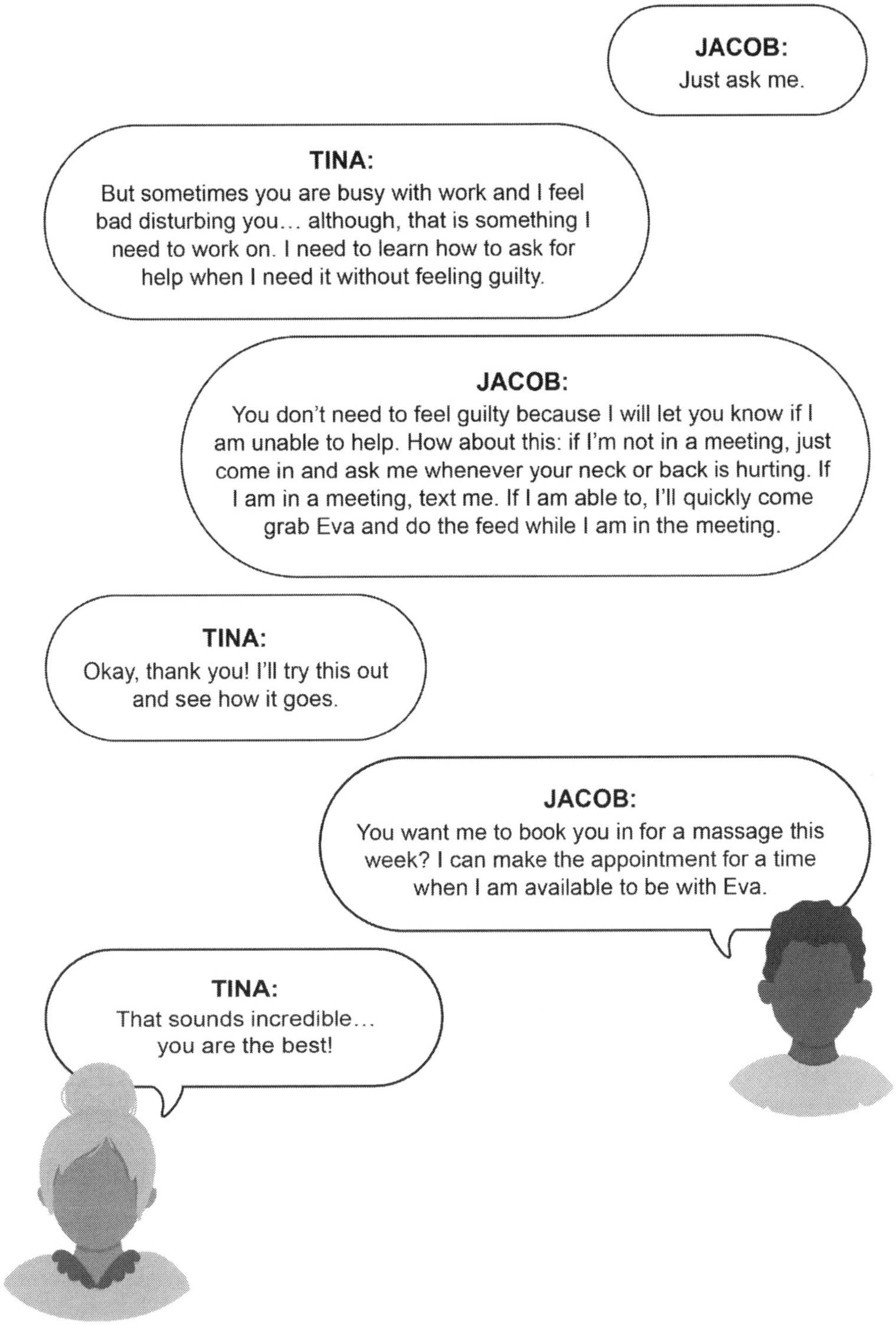
JACOB:
Just ask me.
TINA:
But sometimes you are busy with work and I feel bad disturbing you… although, that is something I need to work on. I need to learn how to ask for help when I need it without feeling guilty.
JACOB:
You don't need to feel guilty because I will let you know if I am unable to help. How about this: if I'm not in a meeting, just come in and ask me whenever your neck or back is hurting. If I am in a meeting, text me. If I am able to, I'll quickly come grab Eva and do the feed while I am in the meeting.
TINA:
Okay, thank you! I'll try this out and see how it goes.
JACOB:
You want me to book you in for a massage this week? I can make the appointment for a time when I am available to be with Eva.
TINA:
That sounds incredible… you are the best!

Similarly, it would be wise to reach out to anyone else you have listed as a source of support to communicate your plan of requesting their help in times of need. Of course, they would have to agree to your plan. While it is unlikely for someone to turn down your request if your plan is communicated with respect and humility, please do manage expectations of your loved ones. Sometimes people's words and actions do not align, in spite of their best intentions.

To demonstrate how you can have a conversation about your care plan with someone other than your partner, I have showcased a dialogue between Amber and Jenny. Amber has a toddler, Greyson, and she is nine months pregnant with her second child. In the following dialogue, she reaches out to her sister-in-law, Jenny, to communicate her care plan and ask for her help:

AMBER:

Hey Jenny! As you know, I am due in a few weeks and I am starting to get a little nervous about how I will manage Greyson and the baby together. I am creating a plan for myself to make sure I have some form of support in place if it gets too much on some days. I'm especially nervous about the days Eric will be traveling for work. Since you live the closest to us, would it be okay for me to drop Greyson off if I am really struggling?

JENNY:

I would love to help you. My concern is that my work is very demanding and my days are usually jam packed with meetings all the way till about 4 PM. How about you drop him off in the evenings whenever you need the help?

AMBER:

Okay, I'll keep that in mind. I have asked my mom for help too but because she lives further away, I thought I'd ask you as well since it might be more convenient to drop him off somewhere closer.

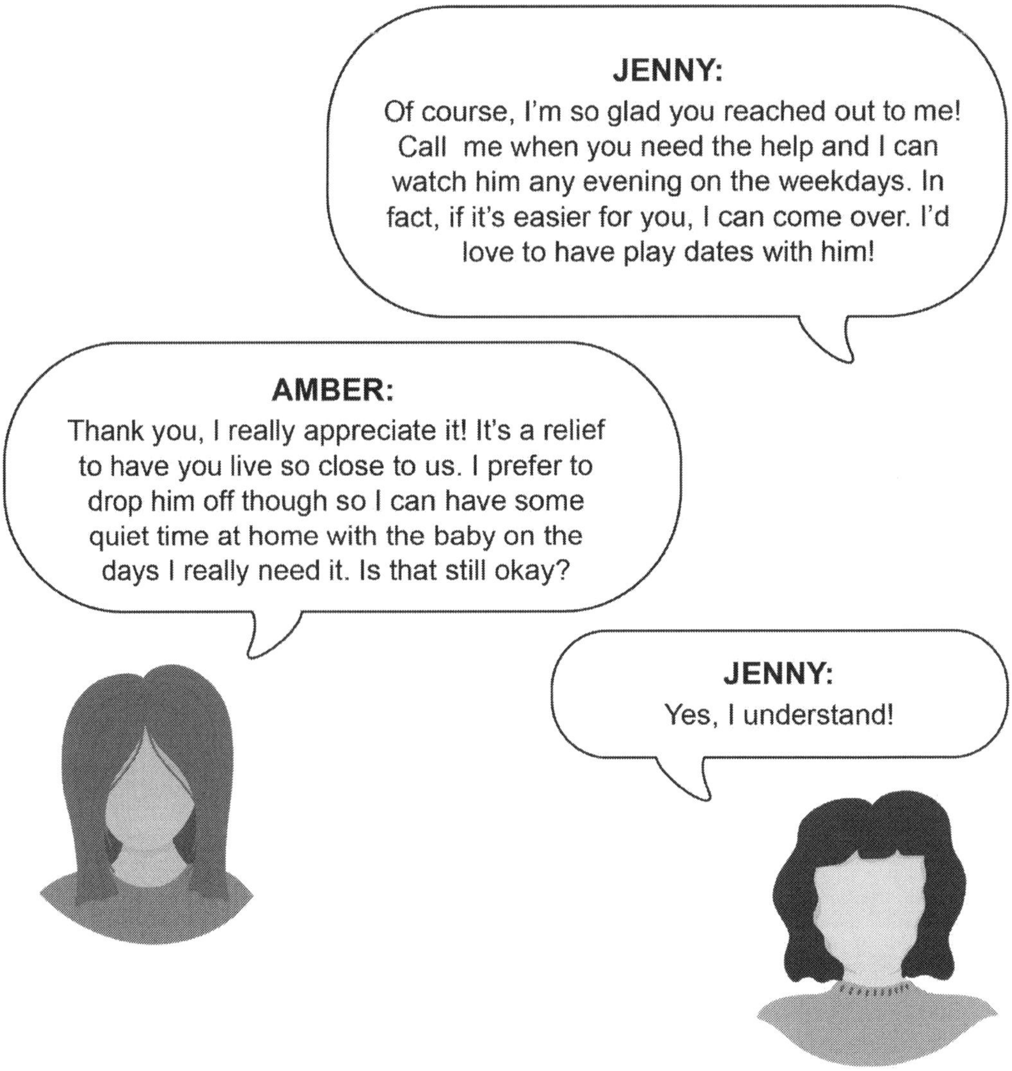
JENNY:
Of course, I'm so glad you reached out to me! Call me when you need the help and I can watch him any evening on the weekdays. In fact, if it's easier for you, I can come over. I'd love to have play dates with him!
AMBER:
Thank you, I really appreciate it! It's a relief to have you live so close to us. I prefer to drop him off though so I can have some quiet time at home with the baby on the days I really need it. Is that still okay?
JENNY:
Yes, I understand!

To demonstrate how you can enlist a friend for support as part of your self-care plan, consider this example:

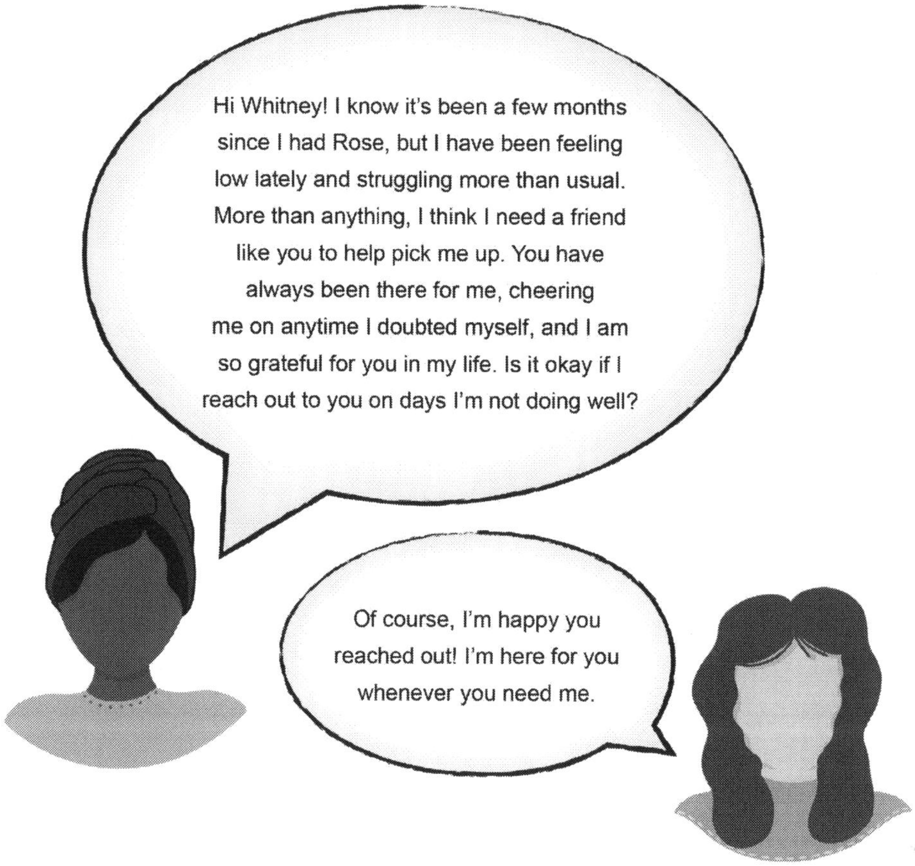
Hi Whitney! I know it's been a few months
since I had Rose, but I have been feeling
low lately and struggling more than usual.
More than anything, I think I need a friend
like you to help pick me up. You have
always been there for me, cheering
me on anytime I doubted myself, and I am
so grateful for you in my life. Is it okay if I
reach out to you on days I'm not doing well?
Of course, I'm happy you
reached out! I'm here for you
whenever you need me.

4. How can you hold someone accountable?

You have created your care plan, communicated it, and received consent from your partner, friends, and family members who have agreed to support you in various ways. But what happens when a person(s) you were expecting support from is not following through with the commitment they made? After all, things can change in a person's life. A family member may no longer be able to help you in the way they initially committed to, a friend may forget, or your partner may be inconsistent with their help.

It might be helpful to have an open, respectful conversation to understand the other person's circumstances and determine whether you need to manage your expectations of them. For example, a conversation may provide clarity to both you and your partner around how they can support you better. It can help you both re-evaluate what seems reasonable and possible now that the baby is here. It can also help you recognize any limitations you didn't take into account when you created your care plan.

Ideally, you have several forms of support listed in your care plan. Here are a few more tips you can consider if a loved one seems to be falling short in providing support in the way you need:

1. Determine whether you clearly communicate your need for help when you need it. Also think about the manner in which you communicate your request.

2. Re-evaluate your expectations. A check-in with a friend or family member can help you assess whether your expectations are exceeding what they are capable of. In this case, you may need to manage your expectations.

3. It might be helpful to use gentle reminders with your loved ones, as needed. For example, you may come to realize that your partner requires a reminder the night before when you are expecting their help with something the following day.

4. If it is someone you have hired for help, such as a babysitter or a nanny, it may be worthwhile to have at least one conversation with them where you respectfully re-assert your expectations before finding someone else for the job.

5. Consider if there is someone else you can ask for help who may be more available or naturally inclined to support you in the manner you need it. Different people in your life will have different strengths; therefore, not everyone will be equally capable of meeting your various needs. Depending on what your need is, whether it is help with performing a task, planning an event, babysitting, or a need for love, connection, reassurance, or any other form of emotional support, consider turning to the person who seems naturally good at offering this type of support.

Prioritizing your physical and mental health is not selfish. To help you understand this, I will share the analogy one of my professors used to explain the importance of self-care: If you have ever been on an airplane, you'll know that flight attendants tell all passengers to put on their own oxygen mask before helping children and other people around them in case of an emergency. The reasoning is, if a passenger does not put on their own mask first, they will start to lose oxygen. This runs the risk of them losing consciousness and not being able to help themselves or others around them who require assistance. Therefore, you are directed to put on your oxygen mask first so you remain conscious and better able to assist those who need help around you.

Being a parent is similar to being a passenger on the plane. You need to be able to take care of yourself first before you can take care of your children. In fact, you will be able to take care of your children better once your own physical and mental health is looked after. And when you start to take care of yourself, parenthood might feel a little less challenging!

Self-care not only benefits you, but it also benefits your family because it makes you proactive, responsible, and wise. While I hope to normalize and encourage self-care for parents, especially the primary parents, I also recognize that not all of you have support in your life. Some of you may be a single parent, living far away from family and friends, have strained relationships, financially unable to hire help, or have a partner who is unable or unwilling to provide you the support you need. I recognize how difficult it might be for you to find a moment to take care of yourself. I sincerely hope by reading this chapter, I have inspired you with an idea or two to try and see if that moment can be made possible. You are worthy of caring for yourself and being cared for by someone else.

Managing Sensory Overload

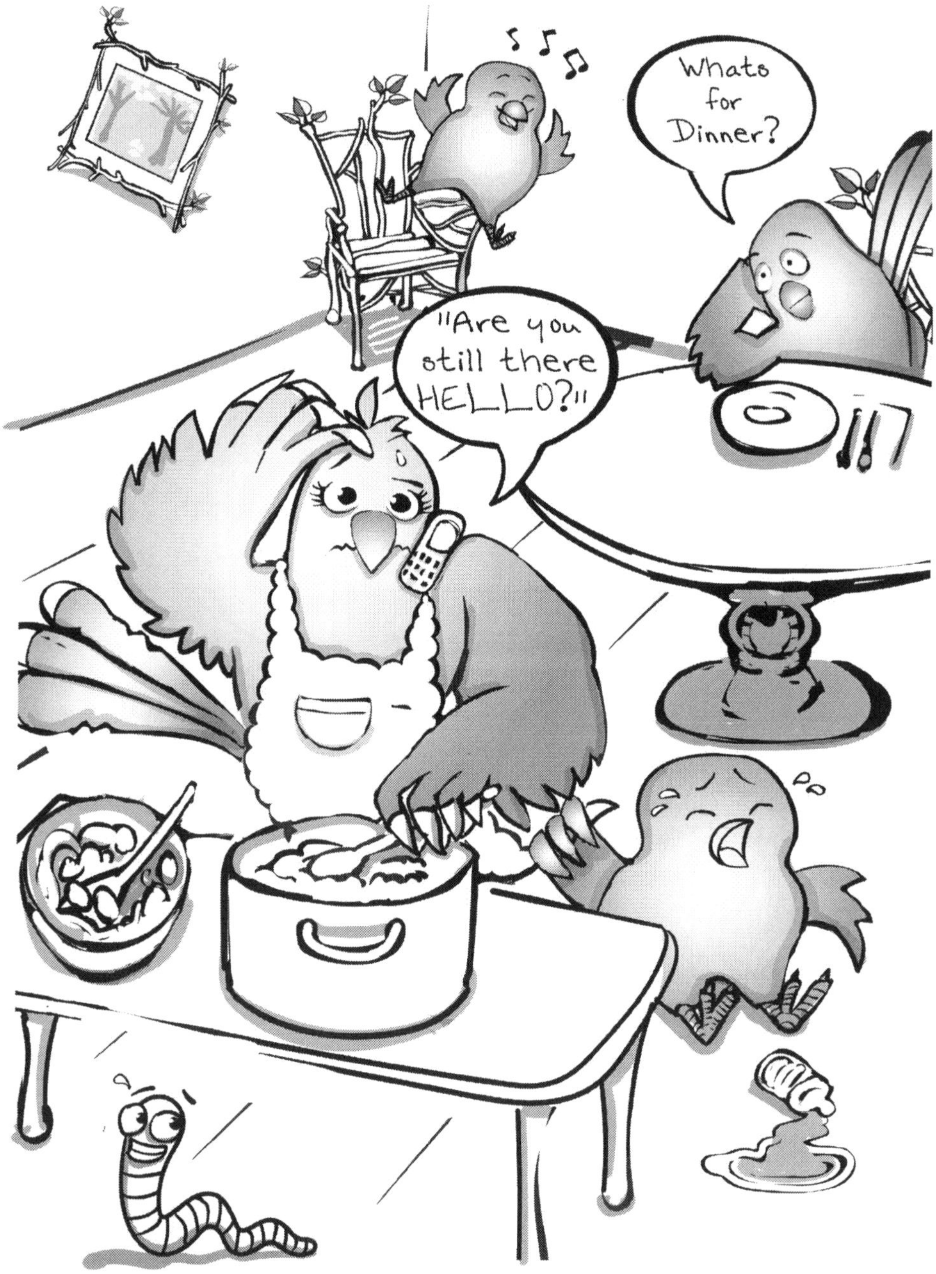
Whats for Dinner?
"Are you still there HELLO?"

With many demands of parenthood competing with each other, it is easy for a parent to feel overstimulated. I have noticed how this can be especially true if you're an anxious person by nature. Because of anxiety, you may be prone to being hypervigilant to visual and auditory cues, making you more susceptible to sensory overload. With all the sounds, visuals, smells, and touch demanding your attention, your brain can activate survival mode, arousing your body to prepare for a threat. In this case, the threat can be as simple as feeling out of control in one too many ways with all the sensory input. Thus, you might start to experience adrenaline rush, muscle tightening, jaw clenching, shallow breathing, inability to pay attention, feeling on edge, and panic.

In response to what your body is experiencing, you might completely shut down, lock yourself in a room to hide somewhere, or feel like running away. Or you might become highly anxious, irritable, and angry enough to scream or rage. It is important to highlight that sleep deprivation, exhaustion, and hunger make matters worse because they reduce your brain's capacity to receive, process, and manage sensory input. As stressed in other parts of this book, this is another reason why it is important to tend to your physical needs.

If any of this sounds like you, please know these are normal experiences when you have small children. During this time, there are many competing demands of life and parenthood. You are not a bad parent for not being able to cope well with sensory overload. However, to ensure your safety and that of your children, it is paramount for you to develop healthy coping skills.

Here are a few techniques to help ground your senses when you are feeling overstimulated:

Sensory Regulation Techniques

01 Breathe

02 Feel

03 Hug

04 Step away

1. **Breathe:** Do a breathing exercise where you imagine creating a square with your breathing. Slowly breathe in from your nose for four counts as you imagine drawing the first line of the square in your mind, filling the air deep into your belly. Next, hold your breath for four counts as you imagine drawing the second line of the box. Then, release the air slowly for four counts from your mouth as you imagine the third line. Finally, hold your breath for four counts as you imagine finishing off the square with the fourth line. You can do this technique as many times as you need until you feel yourself less overwhelmed and more regulated.

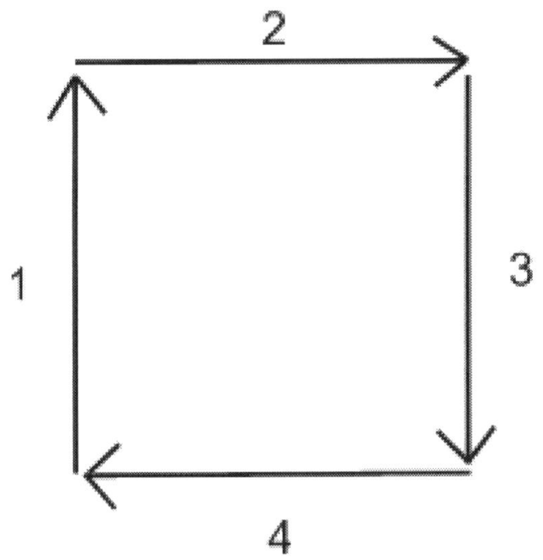
2
1
3
4

2. **Feel:** Use touch as a way to get yourself out of your head and into your body in the present moment. Rub your hands together a few times, as if it's chilly. Next, place your palms on something cold, like the kitchen countertop or a glass window nearby. Pay attention to the cold as it seeps into your palms. If your hands were cold to begin with, touch something warm instead, such as the back of your neck. You can also feel your heartbeat to bring warmth and comfort. Place your hand on your chest and notice your heart beating fast. Breathe slowly and deeply as you do this and notice how your heartbeat slows down. Finally, you can plant your bare feet firmly to the floor to help you ground and anchor yourself quite literally to give you a sense of safety and stability.

3. **Hug:** You can wrap your arms around your chest as if you are holding, hugging, or comforting yourself. You can also ask to be hugged by someone you feel safe with, such as your partner or a family member. Ask for a long hug so you can take comfort in being held by someone you trust and who makes you feel safe.

4. **Step away:** Ask your partner or a support person to step in and be with your children so you can remove yourself from the overly stimulating environment. If you are alone, see if you can put your baby in a safe space, such as their crib with some toys, so you can take a few minutes to be by yourself in a quiet space. Use this time to engage in self-regulation or enlist your partner's help for co-regulation. To review emotion regulation techniques, you can refer back to the sections on page 91 and page 99.

If you find these techniques helpful, you can write them in your self-care plan as coping skills for managing sensory overload. Make sure to practice these techniques every day, even if you are not feeling overstimulated. This will help you determine which techniques are effective for you. More importantly, the more you practice, the easier it will become to rely on these coping skills when you need them the most.

The Stress Response Cycle

Being parents to babies and toddlers perpetually feels like being in survival mode. As a parent, sometimes I find I can't catch a break, jumping from one stressful moment to another. For example, on some mornings there is chaos in my house before I meet my first client of the day for online sessions. Since working from home due to the pandemic, I don't have a commute to allow me the time to transition from parent to professional. Therefore, I have to intentionally carve out time before my first session to release the stress of a challenging morning and transition to my role as a therapist. Before I explain how and why I intentionally release stress, let me first describe how it can build up on a difficult morning:

The first sign of stress begins when I hear my daughter wake up. She is two years old and an early riser—a little too early for my liking. She cries at the crack of dawn (or earlier) every morning until we come to her. Either I or my husband rushes to her room to pick her up from her crib to avoid waking up her brother, who sleeps in the adjacent room. The only way to keep her quiet and settled a little while longer is to bring her to our room and give her milk. That means one of us has to run down to the kitchen and warm up her milk quickly. You see, my daughter hasn't yet learned the virtue of patience.

My son wakes up about an hour later. With all of us awake, I have to move at a steady pace to get my children freshened up, fed, dressed, and out the door with their lunches packed so I can have a few minutes to get myself ready and have a bite to eat before my first session.

A typical morning involves keeping our two children away from each other long enough to keep them focused on getting ready and fed. My children love to be around each other and play together. However, they are both at developmental stages where they want the same thing, and they have trouble sharing. Therefore, there are lots of screams, fights, tantrums, and tears involved. This is why I leave my daughter in our bedroom with my husband while I help my son get ready for the day. However, on these chaotic mornings, my daughter cries for me in the next room while my son takes a *very* long time to complete each task.

Once I finally get my son dressed, I serve him breakfast. I then have to prepare and pack my son's lunch while making my daughter's breakfast at record speed so my husband can come down to begin his work while I go back upstairs to be with my daughter. To remind you, our strategy in the mornings is to keep our children separate—which means one of us has to keep our daughter content and busy separately so her brother remains focused on finishing his breakfast. However, on these challenging mornings, my son has different plans as I find him watching his breakfast instead of eating it. Or I find him playing pretend with invisible cars crashing into each other on the breakfast table.

Once upstairs with my daughter, I might have a moment to pause and think about what I need to do next, but that moment doesn't last long on some mornings. I hear my son running up because he has to use the bathroom, leaving his breakfast unfinished. As he is using the bathroom, my daughter joins him for company if the door is left open.

I stop whatever I'm doing to take her out of the bathroom for fear of what I might discover if I leave her in there. If you're the parent of a toddler, you probably know from experience why leaving them unattended in the bathroom is never a good idea! As I attempt to bring my daughter out, she becomes very upset. As I help her regulate, I realize I need to go back inside to help my son. Now my daughter's crying again and probably banging on the door.

I ask my son to go down to finish his breakfast, but it is too late—he is distracted by his sister. They start running around and playing. I remind my son several times over their playful yelling and excitement that he has to finish his breakfast. Once he finally agrees to go downstairs, I try to get a hold of my daughter to give her breakfast and change her clothes. She loves to run around and get in corners of the house that I have difficulty accessing. I grab a hold of her and attempt to change her clothes as she tries to crawl out of my grip. During this time, she also needs a diaper change. And like many toddlers, she does *not* like to have her diaper changed.

In case you're wondering, my husband and I have a mutual understanding where I look after the kids in the morning so he can begin his work early, and he looks after the drop-offs so I can begin my work on time. Without going into logistical details, this is what works best for both of us to accommodate our work schedules.

As I'm finally able to get ready for work myself, my son and daughter play together for a few minutes. If I'm lucky, they are playing together amicably, and I can focus on myself. With a few minutes left on the clock before my first client, my husband takes my daughter to daycare. At this point, I usually have a back-and-forth exchange with my son where he tries to negotiate for more play time while I remind him about needing to be ready by the door for his dad to take him to school. To speed things up, this requires me to help him put away his toys, put on his sunscreen, his shoes, and his backpack.

As you're reading the events of this morning, you might be able to sense how my stress level remains elevated throughout the morning as I jump from one task to another without having the chance to release my stress in between. This is why I make sure to complete my stress response cycle before I begin my work. That is, I give myself at least 10 minutes to go to my desk and focus on deep breathing to release all the built-up stress in my body. This helps me enter a relaxed state, become present, and feel ready to provide my clients the support they need in online therapy.

The stress response cycle is based on the discoveries of Hans Selye, founder of the stress theory (1946). As illustrated in Figure 15, the stress response cycle begins when your body experiences stress in the face of a perceived threat and ends when your body reaches a state of equilibrium once it realizes it is safe again. In their book, *Burnout: The Secret to Solving the Stress Cycle* (2019), sisters and authors Amelia and Emily Nagoski explain the importance of completing the stress response cycle. They argue that humans tend to live in a constant state of stress without completing the cycle to help their bodies return to a sense of safety.

When you don't engage in a conscious attempt at completing your stress cycle, you don't allow your body to relax. Your body remains in a state of survival mode, facing one stressor after another without having a chance to deactivate the fight, flight, or freeze response. This can leave you feeling on edge, irritable, impatient, reactive, angry, exhausted, and drained, eventually leading to a state of burnout.

Figure 15

Stress response cycle

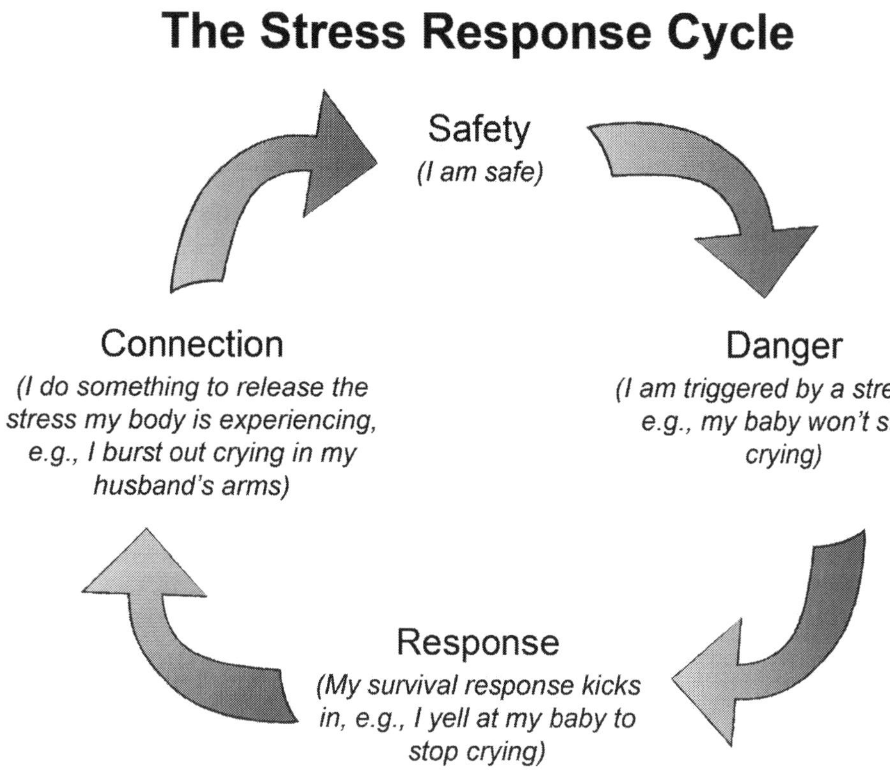
The Stress Response Cycle
Safety
(I am safe)
Danger
(I am triggered by a stressor, e.g., my baby won't stop crying)
Response
(My survival response kicks in, e.g., I yell at my baby to stop crying)
Connection
(I do something to release the stress my body is experiencing, e.g., I burst out crying in my husband's arms)

Note: Original art & material by Zara Arshad, adapted from Janae Elisabeth's "The Stress Cycle Poster" (2020)

This theory resonates with the experiences of many parents with small children, like me. On difficult mornings, I face one stressor after another without having the chance to enter a state of equilibrium. Thus, I make it a point to complete the cycle and release stress from my body through mindfulness once I reach my desk. This helps my body feel safe and connected to the present moment.

The concept of mindfulness was introduced into the Western world by Dr. Jon Kabat-Zinn, founder of the well-known Mindfulness-Based Stress

Reduction Clinic (1979). Dr. Kabat-Zinn teaches you how to use somatic meditation to help you focus on your internal sensations as a way of coping with stress. If you are interested in learning more about mindfulness to help you manage your stress better and live a more stress-free life, I encourage you to read his work. He has written several books, such as *Mindfulness for Beginners* (2016) and *Full Catastrophe Living: Using the Wisdom of Your Body and Mind to Face Stress, Pain and Illness* (2013).

Dr. Peter Levine is also an important figure to note in the field of somatic therapy—a treatment which involves mind and body awareness. Levine, author of *Waking the Tiger, Healing Trauma* (1997), is known for his work on bringing awareness to bodily sensations in order to heal trauma. His approach is based on the theory that the physiological impact of trauma lives inside the body, even after the trauma ends—similar to how stress continues to live in our body even after the stressor(s) ends.

If you sometimes find yourself experiencing one stressor after another without a break, or you feel agitated even after the stressors end, it may benefit you to learn how to complete your stress response cycle. Learning this skill will help you manage your stress better, which will positively influence your physical and mental health, your relationship with your partner, your children, and even yourself. The following are seven evidenced-based techniques suggested by the Nagoski sisters in their book *Burnout: The Secret to Solving the Stress Cycle* (2019):

Tips to Complete Your Stress Cycle

01 Move your body

02 Breathe

03 Cry

04 Laugh

05 Engage in casual social interaction

06 Reach out to a loved one

07 Do something creative

1. **Move your body:** To make the stress hormones dissipate from your body, go for a run, exercise, play a sport, or put on some music and dance! Even pacing is a way of moving your body.
2. **Breathe:** Engage in a deep breathing exercise, such as the square breathing technique on page 280.
3. **Cry:** Let yourself cry for a few minutes. While crying won't necessarily make your situation any better, it will help you feel better because it completes the cycle by releasing the built-up stress from your body.
4. **Laugh:** Laughter—the deep, uncontrollable kind—not only helps people bond but it also helps to ease tension and release happy

hormones in the body. If your partner is the one to make you laugh, go spend some time with them. If it's a friend, make a plan to meet up before the day ends. You can also watch your favorite comedy show, a funny movie, YouTube clips of animals and babies doing silly things, or TikTok videos.

5. **Engage in a casual social interaction:** When you talk to people casually in a social setting, it helps your mind and body perceive the world as a safe, comforting place—a message your body needs to complete the cycle. You can go for a walk and greet people in your neighborhood, go to a local coffee shop and interact with the cashier as you place your order, or strike up a casual conversation with someone as you wait in line at the grocery store.
6. **Reach out to a loved one:** Sometimes, you are too stressed to laugh or engage in small talk. If this is the case, reach out to someone who you love, trust, and feel safe with. This can be any loving and comforting presence in your life, whether it is your partner, parent, sibling, or friend.
7. **Do something creative:** Engaging in a creative activity you enjoy can help you process, express, and release your emotions, including stress. Examples of creative activities include painting, knitting, creating music, graphic design, theater, wood working, and interior decorating.

Along with these tips, if you are a person of faith, engaging with your higher power through prayer or meditation can also provide stress relief. I have presented several techniques you can use to release your stress and complete your stress response cycle. However, not all techniques will be helpful for you. You will need to try them out to see which you find most effective, keeping in mind that different techniques can come in handy during different circumstances.

As a reminder, it is important to give yourself the opportunity to practice so you are ready to use one of the techniques when you need it the most. Assuming you experience at least one stressor in a day, whether it is mild, moderate, or extreme, choose a different technique and practice every day. Practicing consistently will help you develop healthy coping habits to manage your stress and teach you tools to help your mind and body return to a sense of safety.

Reducing Self-Doubt and Guilt

There are many emotions prevalent in motherhood, but the two that gut me every time are self-doubt and guilt. These emotions trumped all others when I had my first child. They were the emotions that led me to question whether I was a good mother, and they contradicted my self-care. I worried and wondered about things such as:

Am I doing enough?

Am I doing something wrong?

Am I unintentionally harming my child's physical or mental health?

Am I still a good wife?

Am I still a good homemaker?

It took me some time to learn these self-doubts are a common part of motherhood, and I was not, in fact, a bad mother just because my guilt was making me believe I was. Like me and the mothers I see in my practice, here are some thoughts you might be having when you are experiencing mom guilt:

- *"I can't believe I yelled at him. I'm a horrible mother."*
- *"I'm ungrateful and don't deserve to be a mother."*
- *"I'm not a good mother if I'm prioritizing my needs over my kids."*
- *"I go to work every day and leave my kids in someone else's care. What kind of a mother am I?"*

- *"I always wanted to be a mother. Why do I feel unhappy?"*
- *"I hate when I don't serve her home-cooked meals. I should be a better mother."*
- *"I can't stay out for long; it would be selfish."*
- *"I can't handle taking care of my kids on my own. I'm always on edge and angry with them. I'm not a fit mother."*
- *"All the other moms seem to be so good at doing arts and crafts and other fun activities with their toddlers at home. Why don't I feel like doing this?"*
- *"It's my fault she got hurt. I should've known better."*
- *"Why can't I breast feed like all the other moms? What's wrong with me?"*

My husband would argue fathers also experience guilt. And he is right, because it is an emotion that can be experienced by both mothers and fathers. In fact, I am well aware of the immense guilt my husband formerly struggled with when he occasionally lost his patience with one of our children.

My husband would withdraw for hours, and sometimes it took him a couple of days to recover as he would become distant and emotionally unavailable to me and our children. I understood his need for space as he needed time to process his anger and the crippling guilt that would take over him. However, that understanding didn't lessen the load on me to 1) step in to repair any damage and make sure my children understood what happened in a way that made sense to them, 2) look after their emotional needs to ensure they felt safe and loved, 3) continue to care for their physical needs alone, 4) be there for my husband to remind him what a loving and caring father he really is, and 5) extend my encouragement and support to him as he learned how to cope with his anger better.

Fortunately, my husband now manages any angry feelings like a champ. What has helped him the most is understanding his internal process by recognizing what triggers his anger and evaluating the purpose of the all-consuming guilt. This self-awareness has helped him manage his stress better, learn to regulate his anger, process any guilt quickly, and use it as a reminder for making repairs with our children right away. By making a repair soon after a rupture, it does wonders to a child's emotional development because it directly feeds into their self-worth. You may recall I discussed an example of a rupture followed by a repair between a parent and a child on page 156.

If you actively work on resolving these feelings, as my husband eventually did, self-doubt and guilt can serve a purpose in helping you re-evaluate and improve your behaviors as a parent. However, these feelings are not necessarily good indicators of the *quality* of your parenting. This is because your internal dialogue about what makes a "good" parent or a "bad" parent is likely based on your subconscious mental images, as I explained earlier in this chapter. For example, when you don't perfectly match your mental image of a "good" parent, you may automatically start engaging in an internal dialogue (your thoughts) full of doubts about yourself as a parent. These doubts can trigger feelings of guilt, anxiety, and depression. Guilt that arises from these negative thought patterns do not serve a purpose beyond making you dislike yourself and leaving you feeling stuck in a negative narrative about yourself and how you relate to your children.

As I shared earlier, I went through a particularly rough postpartum year after my daughter was born. After months of quiet suffering, I made a conscious decision to channel my doubts and guilt into productive behaviors. I no longer wanted to allow these feelings to negatively influence my mood and my self-worth. I now use self-doubts and guilt as indicators to pay attention to my inner dialogue, that is, what I'm saying to myself in my thoughts. I assess whether my doubts are stemming from any subconscious mental images of what a mother should be like. And if they are, I compassionately redirect my thoughts to remember what I *choose* to define as being a good mother.

Regardless of any unconscious images still prevailing in my mind, this is the image of a good mother that I have created consciously:

A good mother is imperfect. She makes mistakes, accepts her limitations, and realizes her strengths. She recognizes that nothing she does from a place of love is going to leave permanent damage. She grows with her children as she learns to parent them. She recognizes the power of making repairs with her children, and she holds herself with compassion while learning from her mistakes and shortcomings. She makes efforts to improve herself as a parent. She focuses more on enjoying moments, creating memories, and living experiences. She does not hyper-focus on a single aspect of her parenting as the be-all, end-all of raising a healthy and secure child. Instead, she has a more holistic view of raising healthy, happy, and secure children. A good mother knows she is enough because she is trying her best every day, and she knows her best may look different every day.

This is my *conscious* definition of a good mother, and it is the one I aspire to. Aligning with this definition has been an important tool in reducing my doubts and guilt, which have become less frequent and less persistent. This definition also teaches me to practice self-compassion, gives me hope, and encourages me to grow with my children and for my children. Self-compassion has been instrumental in allowing me space to breathe as a mother, instead of leaving me stuck in negative thoughts which serve no useful purpose.

Self-compassion is a useful tool in managing self-doubts and guilt. The best way to practice self-compassion is to tell yourself exactly what you would tell a friend or a loved one if they listed out all the reasons why they felt they were a bad mother or father.

What would you say to them?

What would you remind them of?

What tone will you use to convey your thoughts?

How would you want them to feel after speaking with you?

The warmth, grace, and understanding you would want to extend to a loved one is the same warmth, grace, and understanding you want to extend to yourself when you experience guilt. If people you love are worthy of compassion, so are you.

Here is another exercise you can use to increase self-compassion:

Imagine you're carrying a backpack on your shoulders. This backpack is heavy because it is chock full of images, thoughts, ideas, fears, and opinions about what makes a good parent. In the first column, identify and list out as many ideas that automatically come to mind about what being a good parent is. Next, spend some time evaluating which ideas you'd like to keep, and which ones you prefer to throw out (or replace) now that you are looking at them with more awareness.

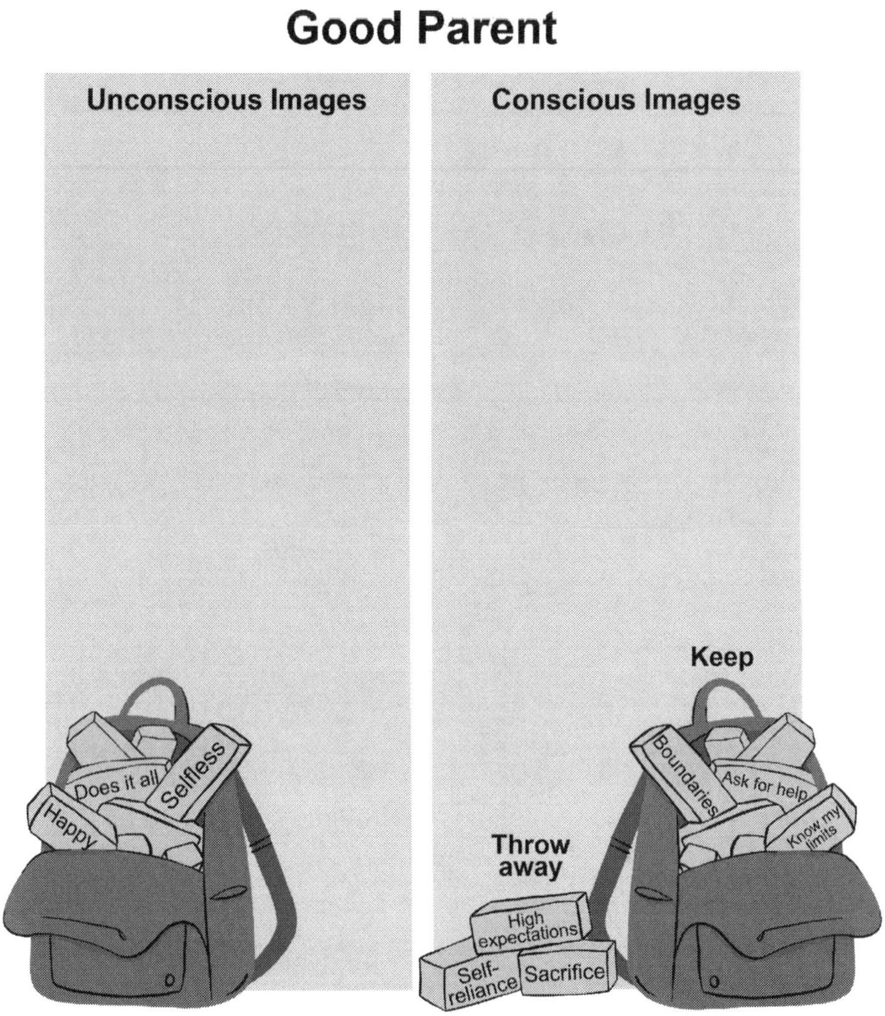
Good Parent
Unconscious Images
Conscious Images
Does it all
Selfless
Happy
Keep
Boundaries
Ask for help
Know my limits
Throw away
High expectations
Self-reliance
Sacrifice

If you're unsure how to evaluate the images and ideas in your good parent backpack, ask yourself the following questions:

- Where did I learn this idea of what a good parent is?
- What purpose is this idea serving in my life as a parent?
- Is this idea leaving me feeling good as a parent, or worse?
- Does this idea leave room for self-compassion?
- Is this idea restrictive or expansive?

- Is this idea creating feelings of doubt and guilt in me?
- What would I say to a friend or a sibling if they shared this idea with me? Would I affirm their idea or would I advise them to modify or replace it?

After you have completed the process of evaluating your subconscious images, ideas, and thoughts, list out which ideas you prefer keeping in the second column, making sure to also brainstorm new ideas you'd like to incorporate in your new definition of a good parent. Images and ideas of a good parent can include spending time with your children, engaging in bonding experiences, self-care, self-compassion, asking for help when you're struggling, regulating your emotions, making repairs, implementing conscious parenting methods, doing your best to serve home-cooked meals, breast or formula feeding, sharing your values, taking interest in your children, being present with them, educating and improving yourself, being emotionally available, balancing a career, taking out time for your interests and hobbies, taking a break, and having good boundaries.

Through this exercise, you can create a framework of what a good parent is to you and learn to make conscious decisions as a parent to help you align to this framework. This tool can teach you how to replace your doubts and guilt with confidence in your capabilities, increase motivation to improve and grow, and have compassion for yourself.

Final Thoughts

As our journey together comes to a close, I want to commend you for finding the time to move through this information. In writing this book, my heartfelt goal was to inspire and encourage couples, new parents, mothers, and fathers. I hope the tools you have learned will support you in your journey ahead as you love and raise your children together. Parenting is not for the faint of heart, and very few of us are given information or a roadmap to help navigate the first year of parenthood.

As you move ahead in your journey, you can feel more confident in understanding yourself, your child, and your partner better if you are in a relationship, marriage, or co-parenting relationship. The roadmap you now have includes:

- Preparing for the arrival of your baby
- Learning how to improve postpartum mood disturbances
- Understanding your attachment style
- Communicating and meeting emotional needs
- Building and maintaining connection in your relationship
- Communication strategies
- Self-care plan, including boundaries and managing expectations
- Strategies to navigate common postpartum challenges as a couple

As you review all that you have learned, I hope you are giving yourself a well-deserved pat on the back for taking time to learn how to build a healthy foundation for your children. If you haven't done so, I encourage you to take some time in the reflection sections of this book and add your thoughts while they are fresh in your mind.

Finally, if you are feeling overwhelmed with everything you already have on your plate, wondering how you will apply all that you have learned from this book, be gentle with yourself. Know that you are fully equipped and capable of moving forward and practicing the tools you have learned. It might not feel easy, but it is worth trying!

The reflection sections can serve as your go-to, summarized action plan—and you can take one action at a time. Create your own pace but make sure to keep taking steps and practicing. Practice doesn't make perfect because there is no such thing as a perfect parent or a perfect partner. However, practice creates progress and honors your sincere efforts—every small step you take counts towards something bigger.

If you find you need additional support after reading this book and would like to attend my workshop series, I would love to have you join us. You can learn more about the workshop on my website: https://myottawatherapist.com. You are also welcome to reach out to me through my website for booking an appointment.

In the next and final chapter of this book, I've included several helpful resources to support each and every couple and parent. Please feel free to review and highlight the resources that stand out to you.

I wish you, your relationship, and your baby all the best!

Warmly,

Zara

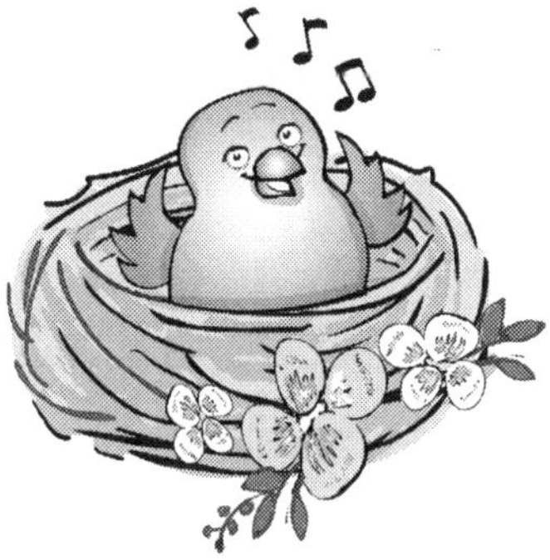

Reflections

What resonated for you in this chapter?

What are the key points you want to remember?

What might be worth discussing with your partner?

What tool or strategy do you want to put into practice?

Chapter 6: *Resources*

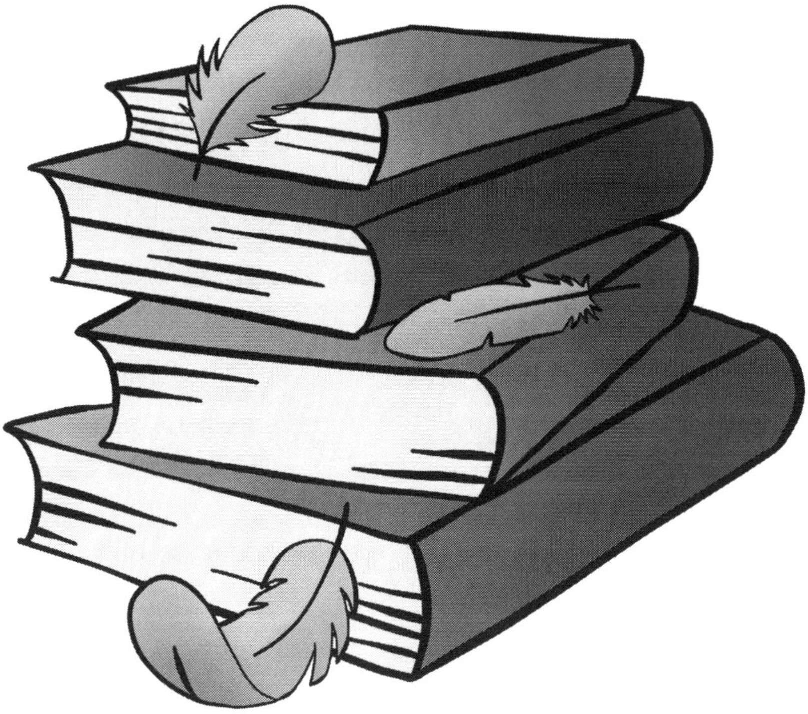

I wrote this book with the intention of empowering readers like you to understand yourself and your relationship better and learn how to navigate life after having a baby. I am aware some readers may require more help and resources to support their relationship and their mental health. It is important for you to recognize your limits and reach out for help when you need it. I have outlined the following resources as additional support.

Medical Professional

Consider consulting with your family doctor as your first point of contact if you are experiencing prolonged or unusual issues during your physical recovery after birth or struggling with anything related to your body. If you feel uncertain about something, it is better to be safe and consult with a professional to rule out any serious issue or prevent the onset of something worse. Your obstetrician and gynecologist will also be a good resource to contact if you have any questions or concerns about your body during your physical recovery. Concerns related to pain from breastfeeding should also be consulted with a doctor or a lactation consultant. A professional can provide you with helpful recommendations to reduce your pain and manage any other symptoms.

Mental Health Professional

If you are experiencing mental health concerns, such as anxiety, depression, frequent feelings of overwhelm, inability to cope with your thoughts and emotions, difficulty in managing daily activities, difficulty in caring for your baby, or distress in relationships with your partner or loved ones, I urge you to book an appointment with a mental health professional. A good place to start is to consult with a local psychotherapist. Chances are a few sessions with an experienced and competent psychotherapist who works with couples and new parents are sufficient in providing you the support and tools needed to improve your mental health and the relationships around you. Sometimes, your psychotherapist may refer you to a psychologist or psychiatrist for an assessment to determine whether you may benefit from a specialized treatment plan and/or medication.

Here are three resources for finding a psychotherapist:

- *Psychology Today*: www.psychologytoday.com
- Postpartum Support International: https://psidirectory.com/
- Your local search engine, such as www.google.com

Medication

While new parenthood is a joyous time for many parents, it can also be a challenging time for most. For some new parents, their transition to parenthood may take a greater toll on their mental health where their ability to tolerate stressors decreases significantly compared to other new parents. For example, if a new parent is hyper-sensitive to stimulations in their environment, if they are quick to be drastically dysregulated when triggered, if they find it difficult to regulate their emotions more than others, if they are unable to sleep or stay asleep at night, or if they have an underlying mental health condition, their window of tolerance may become narrower than others, making it difficult for them to implement what they gain from sessions with their therapist. For these individuals, medication may be necessary in conjunction with talk therapy to help increase their window of tolerance long enough to absorb the benefits of therapy and create long-lasting change.

If you suspect you require medication in conjunction with talk therapy, consult with your therapist and your doctor or psychiatrist to determine what is the best treatment approach for you. It is important to note the decision to start or stop taking medication for mental health concerns needs to be an ongoing discussion between you and all of your health care providers such as your family doctor, psychiatrist, and psychotherapist. In some cases, long-term or life-long use of medication is necessary to manage a clinically diagnosed mental illness and maintain control of the symptoms throughout a person's lifetime.

Infertility and Support Groups

Educating yourself on the topic of infertility using credible sources can increase your knowledge, provide answers, help make sense of your situation, and assist in formulating a plan with your partner to manage issues related to infertility, trauma, and sexual health. I have provided a list of resources which you can use to become more informed. Some of these resources can also be used to locate a support group if you are experiencing poor mental health, loss, and/or grief:

- Fertility Matters Canada: https://fertilitymatters.ca/
- The National Infertility Association: https://resolve.org/
- American Society for Reproductive Medicine: https://www.asrm.org/
- National Library of Medicine: https://www.nlm.nih.gov/
- Postpartum Support International: https://psidirectory.com/

Crisis Hotlines

Your safety and that of your child(ren) is of utmost importance. If you have concerns about suicide, self-harm, harm to another person such as your child, your physical safety, a mental health crisis, being in an abusive relationship, and/or being in any kind of immediate danger, please call 911, a local crisis line, or a local shelter for victims of domestic violence.

I have provided crisis, suicide, domestic violence, and child abuse hotlines in Canada and the United States. If you reside in a different country, please contact a local emergency or crisis service to ensure safety for yourself and your child(ren).

Canada

- Crisis Line
  Call 1-800-668-6868 or text CONNECT 686868

- Talk Suicide
  Call 1-833-456-4566 or text 45645
  https://talksuicide.ca/

- Shelter Safe
  https://sheltersafe.ca/

- Kids Help Phone
  Call 1-800-668-6868 or text to CONNECT 686868
  https://kidshelpphone.ca/

United States

- Crisis Text Line
  Text HOME to 741741
  https://www.crisistextline.org/

- National Suicide and Crisis Lifeline
  Call 988
  https://988lifeline.org/

- National Domestic Violence Hotline
  Call 1-800-799-7233
  https://www.thehotline.org/

- Childhelp National Child Abuse Hotline
  Call or text 1-800-422-4453
  https://childhelphotline.org/

Books

Self-help books are great for increasing your knowledge, understanding, and motivation, as well as for providing tools which can help you begin the process of growth and self-improvement. However, books are limited in their ability to help you create long-lasting changes. I recommend using a self-help book as a starting point for improving yourself and/or your relationship or using it to supplement your work in therapy. Please remember books do not provide the same benefits of therapy; therefore, they should not be used as a replacement for therapy.

These are some of the books I share with clients in my own practice, and the list also includes books my clients have shared with me as being helpful:

Self-improvement

- *Homecoming: Reclaiming and Healing Your Inner Child* by John Bradshaw
- *How to Do the Work: Recognize Your Patterns, Heal from Your Past, and Create Your Self* by Nicole LePera
- *It Didn't Start with You: How Inherited Family Trauma Shapes Who We Are and How to End the Cycle* by Mark Wolynn
- *Rewire Your Brain: Think Your Way to a Better Life* by John B. Arden
- *The Body Keeps the Score: Brain, Mind, and Body in the Healing of Trauma* by Bessel van der Kolk
- *The Power of Vulnerability: Teachings of Authenticity, Connection, and Courage* by Brene Brown
- *To Have and to Hold: Motherhood, Marriage, and the Modern Dilemma* by Molly Millwood
- *Self-Compassion: The Proven Power of Being Kind to Yourself* by Kristin Neff

Relationship Improvement

- *Attached: The New Science of Adult Attachment and How It Can Help You Find—and Keep—Love* by Amir Levine & Rachel Heller
- *Wired for Love: How Understanding Your Partner's Brain and Attachment Style Can Help You Defuse Conflict and Build a Secure Relationship* by Stan Tatkin
- *The 5 Love Languages: The Secret to Love that Lasts* by Gary Chapman
- *The Seven Principles for Making Marriage Work: A Practical Guide from the Country's Foremost Relationship Expert* by John Gottman
- *Hold Me Tight: Seven Conversations for a Lifetime of Love* by Sue Johnson
- *Eight Dates: Essential Conversations for a Lifetime of Love* by John Gottman
- *Us: Getting Past You and Me to Build a More Loving Relationship* by Terrence Real

Parenting

- *Parenting from the Inside Out: How a Deeper Self-Understanding Can Help You Raise Children Who Thrive* by Daniel J. Siegel & Mary Hartzell
- *The Whole-Brain Child: 12 Revolutionary Strategies to Nurture Your Child's Developing Mind* by Daniel Siegel & Tina Payne Bryson
- *Conscious Parenting: A Guide to Raising Resilient, Wholehearted & Empowered Kids* by Pedram Shojai & Nick Polizzi
- *Raising Good Humans: A Mindful Guide to Breaking the Cycle of Reactive Parenting and Raising Kind, Confident Kids* by Hunter Clarke-Fields & Carla Naumburg
- *The Conscious Parent: Transforming Ourselves, Empowering Our Children* by Shefali Tsabary

- *How Not to Hate Your Husband After Kids* by Jancee Dunn
- *Fair Play: A Game-Changing Solution for When You Have Too Much to Do (and More Life to Live)* by Eve Rodsky

Co-Parenting

- *Parenting Apart: How Separated and Divorced Parents Can Raise Happy and Secure Kids* by Christina McGhee
- *Healthy Children of Divorce in 10 Simple Steps: Minimize the Effects of Divorce on Your Children* by Shannon Rios Paulsen
- *The Co-Parenting Handbook: Raising Well-Adjusted and Resilient Kids from Little Ones to Young Adults through Divorce or Separation* by Karen Bonnell
- *Joint Custody with a Jerk: Raising a Child with an Uncooperative Ex* by Julie A. Ross & Judy Corcoran

Social Media

I have found social media spaces, such as Instagram and Facebook, to be good sources of support in that you never feel alone. There is always someone out there going through what you are going through. It helps to create a sense of belonging and connection with other mothers and fathers who are also facing pregnancy and postpartum challenges and trying to navigate their life after birth. Finding people like yourself experiencing similar challenges can bring comfort, relief, patience, and hope for new parents.

Social media also makes it possible for you to directly access the expertise of professionals in the field of mental health, relationships, medicine, perinatal care, and parenting. Finding expert knowledge, tools, and recommendations at your fingertips is remarkable. However, this level of accessibility to information on social media should be consumed cautiously, and with a critical eye. While there is a lot of good information posted on social media, there is also the presence of misinformation and personal opinions presented as facts. Make sure to do your due diligence and consume information from only those accounts that are run by verified, accredited, and licensed professionals. Finally, be mindful of how you utilize social media; it can be beneficial as an additional resource, but it is not a replacement for therapy. Treat social media as a starting point, and not the final stop.

There are many Instagram accounts run by established professionals in their respective fields. While I have put together the following list of accounts for you, please do your due diligence and verify the authenticity and credentials of the person before following their advice:

Self-Improvement

- @the.couples.couch
- @the.holistic.psychologist
- @millennial.therapist
- @doodledwellness
- @attachmentnerd

Relationship

- @the.couples.couch
- @thesecurerelationship
- @couples.counseling.for.parents
- @loveafterbaby
- @drlaurenfogelmersy
- @stephanie__rigg
- @lizlistens

Pregnancy, Birth, and Breastfeeding

- @painfreebirth
- @labor.nurse.mama
- @thelabormama
- @themilknest
- @breastfeeding.dietician

Postpartum

- @happyasamother
- @psychedmommy

Parenting

- @consciousmommy
- @transformingtoddlerhood
- @mellowmama
- @biglittlefeelings
- @ourmamavillage
- @mamapsychologists

Websites and Blogs

It is astounding how you can find any amount of information, knowledge, research, opinions, and subjective experiences on nearly any topic within moments on the Internet. As with social media, I believe the Internet is a good starting point, but it should not be your final stop. Reading through blogs and articles can help you discover and learn something relevant, make sense of something, not feel alone or scared in your experience of something, and help you determine whether you need to continue digging deeper into something. At the same time, reading only blogs and articles runs the risk of leaving you convinced of information presented by non-experts.

If you come across something that seems to answer your question or concern, cross reference it with more credible sources on the Internet, such as research-based findings and articles written by professionals in the field. Additionally, check in with your family doctor, specialist, psychotherapist, midwife, lactation consultant, or another expert who specializes in the area of concern.

I occasionally write about topics related to therapy, couples, and new parents on my blog. If you are interested in reading about these topics and learning some tips along the way, you can follow my blog, *All Things Couples*, on my website: www.myottawatherapist.com.

There are also websites specializing in articles on perinatal topics which provide a wealth of information to expecting couples and parents. These websites also have applications which can be downloaded on your phone. Within the applications, you can find online communities for mothers and fathers which help connect parents from all over the world. Parents share their struggles, ask questions, support each other, share ideas, and provide advice from personal experiences.

These online communities, while not guaranteed to be a safe space, can help provide a sense of belonging, normalcy, and support to couples and single parents. Here are popular ones which you might already be familiar with:

- What to Expect: https://www.whattoexpect.com/
- Baby Center: https://www.babycenter.ca/ and https://www.babycenter.com/
- The Bump: https://www.thebump.com/

Workshops

After reading this book, if you think it would be helpful to have additional support on improving your relationship and managing postpartum challenges, I encourage you to attend one of my workshops for couples and new parents. In these workshops, I help you gain insight into your relationship patterns, increase self-awareness, learn how to improve various aspects of your relationship, and learn tools to manage common postpartum issues. If you are interested in signing up for a workshop, please visit my website: https://www.myottawatherapist.com.

Works Cited

Amankwaa, L. C. (2005). Maternal postpartum role collapse as a theory of postpartum depression. *The Qualitative Report, 10*(1), 21-38. https://doi.org/10.46743/2160-3715/2005.1856

American Psychiatric Association. (2013). *Diagnostic and statistical manual of mental disorders* (5th ed.). https://doi.org/10.1176/appi.books.9780890425596

Bandura, A. (1991). Social cognitive theory of self-regulation. *Organizational Behavior and Human Decision Processes, 50*(2), 248-287. https://doi.org/10.1016/0749-5978(91)90022-L

Barrett, G., Pendry, E., Peacock, J., Victor, C., Thakar, R., & Manyonda, I. (2000). Women's sexual health after childbirth. *International Journal of Obstetrics and Gynaecology, 107*(2), 186–195. https://doi.org/10.1111/j.1471-0528.2000.tb11689.x

Bartellas, E., Crane, J. M., Daley, M., Bennett, K. A., & Hutchens, D. (2000). Sexuality and sexual activity in pregnancy. *International Journal of Obstetrics and Gynaecology, 107*(8), 964–968. https://doi.org/10.1111/j.1471-0528.2000.tb10397.x

Beck, J. S. (2020). *Cognitive behavior therapy* (3rd ed.). Guilford Press.

Bodenmann, G. (1995). A systemic-transactional conceptualization of stress and coping in couples. *Swiss Journal of Psychology, 54*(1), 34–39.

Bodenmann, G., Pihet, S., & Kayser, K. (2006). The relationship between dyadic coping and marital quality: A 2-year longitudinal study. *Journal of family psychology: JFP: journal of the Division of Family Psychology of the American Psychological Association (Division 43), 20*(3), 485–493. https://doi.org/10.1037/0893-3200.20.3.485

Bowlby, J. (1958). The nature of the child's tie to his mother. *The International Journal of Psychoanalysis, 39*(5), 350-373.

Bowlby, J., Ainsworth, M. D., Boston, M., Rosenbluth, D. (1956). Effects of mother-child separation: A follow-up study. *British Journal of Medical Psychology, 29*(3-4), 169-201. https://doi.org/10.1111/j.2044-8341.1956.tb00915.x

Brumariu, L.E. (2015). Parent-Child Attachment and Emotion Regulation. *New Directions for Child and Adolescent Development*, 31-45. https://doi.org/10.1002/cad.20098

Bushnik, T., Cook, J. L., Yuzpe, A. A., Tough, S., & Collins, J. (2012). Estimating the prevalence of infertility in Canada. *Human Reproduction (Oxford, England), 27*(3), 738–746. https://doi.org/10.1093/humrep/der465

Butler, E.A., & Randall, A.K. (2013). Emotional coregulation in close relationships. *Emotion Review, 5*(2), 202–210. https://doi.org/10.1177/175407391245163

Cooney, G. M., Dwan, K., Greig, C. A., Lawlor, D. A., Rimer, J., Waugh, F. R., McMurdo, M., & Mead, G. E. (2013). Exercise for depression. *The Cochrane database of systematic reviews*, (9). https://doi.org/10.1002/14651858.CD004366.pub6

Davidova, K., & Pechova, O. (2014). Infertility and assisted reproduction technologies through a gender lens. *Human Affairs, 24*, 363–375. doi:10.2478/s13374-014-0234-9.

Doss, B. D., Rhoades, G. K., Stanley, S. M., & Markman, H. J. (2009). The effect of the transition to parenthood on relationship quality: An 8-year prospective study. *Journal of Personality and Social Psychology, 96*(3), 601–619. https://doi.org/10.1037/a0013969

Elisabeth, J. (2020, March 2). *The stress cycle poster*. Trauma Geek. https://www.traumageek.com/infographics/the-stress-cycle-poster-pdf-instant-download

Falconier, M. K., Randall, A. K., & Bodenmann, G. (Eds.). (2016). *Couples coping with stress: A cross-cultural perspective*. Routledge/Taylor & Francis Group.

Fernández-Carrasco, F.J., Rodríguez-Díaz, L., González-Mey, U., Vázquez-Lara, J.M., Gómez-Salgado, J., & Parrón-Carreño, T. (2020). Changes in sexual desire in women and their partners during pregnancy. *Journal of Clinical Medicine, 9*(2), 526. https://doi.org/10.3390/jcm9020526

Ghaedrahmati, M., Kazemi, A., Kheirabadi, G., Ebrahimi, A., & Bahrami, M. (2017). Postpartum depression risk factors: A narrative review. *Journal of education and health promotion, 6*(60). https://doi.org/10.4103/jehp.jehp_9_16

Gottman, J. M., & Silver, N. (2000). *The seven principles for making marriage work*. [Pbk. ed.]. New York: Three Rivers Press.

Grewen, K.M., Girdler, S.S., Amico, J., & Light, K.C. (2005). Effects of partner support on resting oxytocin, cortisol, norepinephrine, and blood pressure before and after warm partner contact. *Journal of Biobehavioral Medicine, 67*(4), 531-538. https://doi.org/10.1097/01.psy.0000170341.88395.47

Gutzeit, O., Levy, G., & Lowenstein, L. (2020). Postpartum female sexual function: Risk factors for postpartum sexual dysfunction. *Sexual Medicine*, *8*(1), 8–13. https://doi.org/10.1016/j.esxm.2019.10.005

Jayakody, K., Gunadasa, S., and Horner, C. (2013) Exercise for anxiety disorders: Systematic review. *British Journal of Sports Medicine, 48*(3), 187–196. https://doi.org/10.1136/bjsports-2012-091287

Johnson, S.M. (2004). *The practice of emotionally focused couples therapy: Creating connection* (A.M. Salvetti, Trans.; 2nd ed.). Routledge.

Johnson, S. M., Makinen, J. A., & Millikin, J. W. (2001). Attachment injuries in couple relationships: a new perspective on impasses in couples therapy. *Journal of Marital and Family Therapy*, *27*(2), 145–155. https://doi.org/10.1111/j.1752-0606.2001.tb01152.x

Kabat-Zinn, J. (2012). *Mindfulness for beginners*: *Reclaiming the present moment—and your life*. Boulder, Colorado, Sounds True.

Kabat-Zinn, J. (2013). *Full catastrophe living: Using the wisdom of your body and mind to face stress, pain, and illness*. New York: Bantam Books.

Kotlar, B., Gerson, E., Petrillo, S., Langer, A., & Tiemeier, H. (2021). The impact of the COVID-19 pandemic on maternal and perinatal health: A scoping review. *Reproductive Health*, *18*(1), 10. https://doi.org/10.1186/s12978-021-01070-6

Levine, P. A. (1997). *Waking the tiger: healing trauma: The innate capacity to transform overwhelming experiences*. Berkeley, California: North Atlantic Books.

Kabat-Zinn, Jon. (2013). *Full catastrophe living: Using the wisdom of your body and mind to face stress, pain, and illness.* New York: Bantam Books.

Maslow, A.H. (1943). A theory of human motivation. *Psychological Review, 50*(4), 430-437.

McDonald, E., Woolhouse, H., & Brown, S. J. (2017). Sexual pleasure and emotional satisfaction in the first 18 months after childbirth. *Midwifery, 55,* 60–66. https://doi.org/10.1016/j.midw.2017.09.002

Merriam-Webster. (n.d.). Vulnerable. In *Merriam-Webster.com dictionary.* Retrieved July 20, 2022, from https://www.merriam-webster.com/dictionary/vulnerable

Minuchin, S. (1974). *Families and family therapy.* London: Routledge.

Molgora, S., Fenaroli, V., Acquati, C., De Donno, A., Baldini, M. P., & Saita, E. (2019). Examining the role of dyadic coping on the marital adjustment of couples undergoing assisted reproductive technology (ART). *Frontiers in Psychology, 10,* 415. https://doi.org/10.3389/fpsyg.2019.00415

Nagoski, E. & Nagoski, A. (2019). Burnout: The secret to unlocking the stress cycle. New York: Ballantine Books.

Ninivaggio, C., Rogers, R. G., Leeman, L., Migliaccio, L., Teaf, D., & Qualls, C. (2017). Sexual function changes during pregnancy. *International Urogynecology Journal, 28*(6), 923–929. https://doi.org/10.1007/s00192-016-3200-8

Peterson, B. D., Pirritano, M., Christensen, U., & Schmidt, L. (2008). The impact of partner coping in couples experiencing infertility. *Human Reproduction (Oxford, England)*, *23*(5), 1128–1137. https://doi.org/10.1093/humrep/den067

Rockliff, H. E., Lightman, S. L., Rhidian, E., Buchanan, H., Gordon, U., & Vedhara, K. (2014). A systematic review of psychosocial factors associated with emotional adjustment in in vitro fertilization patients. *Human Reproduction Update*, *20*(4), 594–613. https://doi.org/10.1093/humupd/dmu010

Sauvé, M. S., Péloquin, K., & Brassard, A. (2020). Moving forward together, stronger, and closer: An interpretative phenomenological analysis of marital benefits in infertile couples. *Journal of Health Psychology*, *25*(10-11), 1532–1542. https://doi.org/10.1177/1359105318764283

Schwenck, G. C., Dawson, S. J., Muise, A., & Rosen, N. O. (2020). A comparison of the sexual well-being of new parents with community couples. *The Journal of Sexual Medicine*, *17*(11), 2156–2167. https://doi.org/10.1016/j.jsxm.2020.08.011

Segre, L.S. & Davis, W.N. (2013). *Postpartum Depression and Perinatal Mood Disorders in the DSM*. Postpartum Support International. https://www.postpartum.net/wp-content/uploads/2014/11/DSM-5-Summary-PSI.pdf

Selye, H. (1946). The general adaptation syndrome and the diseases of adaptation. *The Journal of Clinical Endocrinology and Metabolism*, *6*, 117–230. https://doi.org/10.1210/jcem-6-2-117

Shapiro, A.F., Gottman, J.M., & Carrère, S. (2000). The baby and the marriage: Identifying factors that buffer against decline in marital satisfaction after the first baby arrives. *Journal of Family Psychology, 14*(1), 59-70. https://doi.org/10.1037//0893-3200.14.1.59

Signorello, L. B., Harlow, B. L., Chekos, A. K., & Repke, J. T. (2001). Postpartum sexual functioning and its relationship to perineal trauma: A retrospective cohort study of primiparous women. *American Journal of Obstetrics and Gynecology, 184*(5), 881–890. https://doi.org/10.1067/mob.2001.113855

Statistics Canada. (2019). *Maternal Mental Health in Canada, 2019* [Infographic]. https://www150.statcan.gc.ca/n1/pub/11-627-m/11-627-m2019041-eng.pdf

Urlichs, J. (2020). Finding us. *From one mom to a mother* (pp. 65-66). New Zealand: Jessica Urlichs.

Van Anders, S. M., Hipp, L. E., & Kane Low, L. (2013). Exploring co-parent experiences of sexuality in the first 3 months after birth. *The Journal of Sexual Medicine, 10*(8), 1988–1999. https://doi.org/10.1111/jsm.12194

Vigod, S. N., Brown, H. K., Huang, A., Fung, K., Barker, L. C., Hussain-Shamsy, N., Wright, E., Dennis, C. L., Grigoriadis, S., Gozdyra, P., Corsi, D., Walker, M., & Moineddin, R. (2021). Postpartum mental illness during the COVID-19 pandemic: a population-based, repeated cross-sectional study. *Canadian Medical Association journal 193*(23), 835–843. https://doi.org/10.1503/cmaj.210151

Weitkamp, K., Feger, F., Landolt, S. A., Roth, M., & Bodenmann, G. (2021). Dyadic Coping in Couples Facing Chronic Physical Illness: A Systematic Review. *Frontiers in psychology, 12*, 722740. https://doi.org/10.3389/fpsyg.2021.722740

Bio

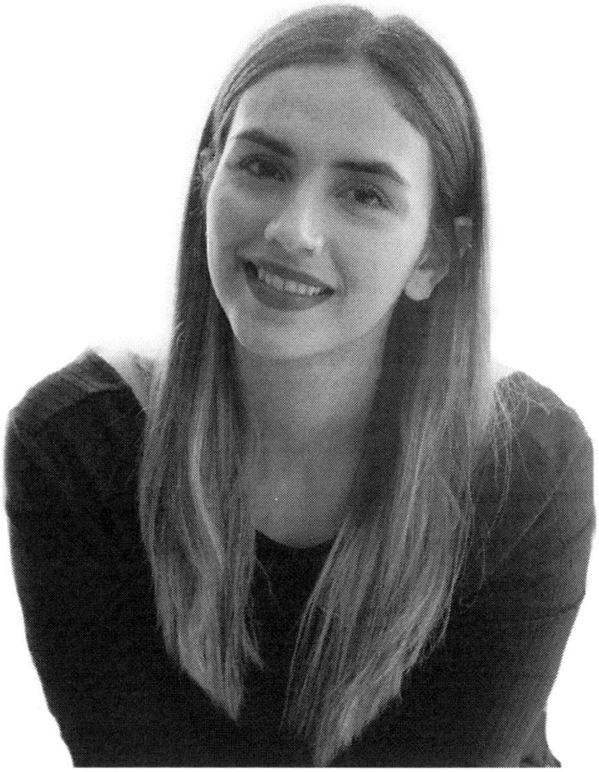

Zara Arshad, born 1989, spent her childhood in Karachi, Pakistan as the youngest in a large family. She moved to Virginia, U.S.A., in 2001 where she eventually earned a Master of Science in Human Development and received professional training as a marriage and family therapist (MFT) from Virginia Polytechnic Institute & State University. While pursuing her masters, she met her fiancé, who she married in 2013. Upon completion of her training in 2015, she moved to Ottawa, ON to be with her husband.

During her time settling in Ottawa, Zara became a published author of a chapter in the book *Couples Coping with Stress: A Cross Cultural Perspective* (2016). Soon after becoming a registered psychotherapist (RP) in Ontario in 2017, she founded "My Ottawa Therapist" (www.myottawatherapist.com), a thriving private practice where she specializes in supporting couples who are dealing with relationship distress and who want to improve their communication, connection, and ability to navigate their relationship postpartum. She also offers workshops (https://www.myottawatherapist.com) to empower couples by helping them understand themselves better as they learn to work through common relationship issues, such as unhealthy communication patterns.

In her personal life, Zara is a dedicated wife to her loving husband and a devoted mother to her two precious children. Zara loves to travel, experience different cultures, visit local coffee shops and antique stores, people watch, read historical fiction, sit by the ocean, soak in the sun, and spend time with family and friends.

Made in the USA
Middletown, DE
12 August 2024

58979700R00196